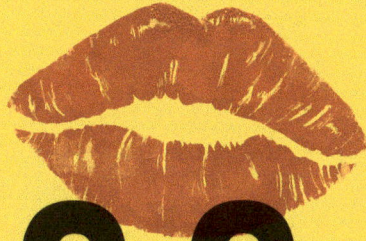

K.I.S.S.

KEEP IT SHORT AND SIMPLE

FOR A HEALTHY, SUSTAINABLE LIFESTYLE

Includes Healthy Recipes, Easy-to-Follow Workouts, and Mindset Training

THE ULTIMATE GUIDE FOR LIVING A HEALTHY, WELL-BALANCED LIFE

DR. TRINA WIGGINS

Over 32 years of practicing medicine & wellness

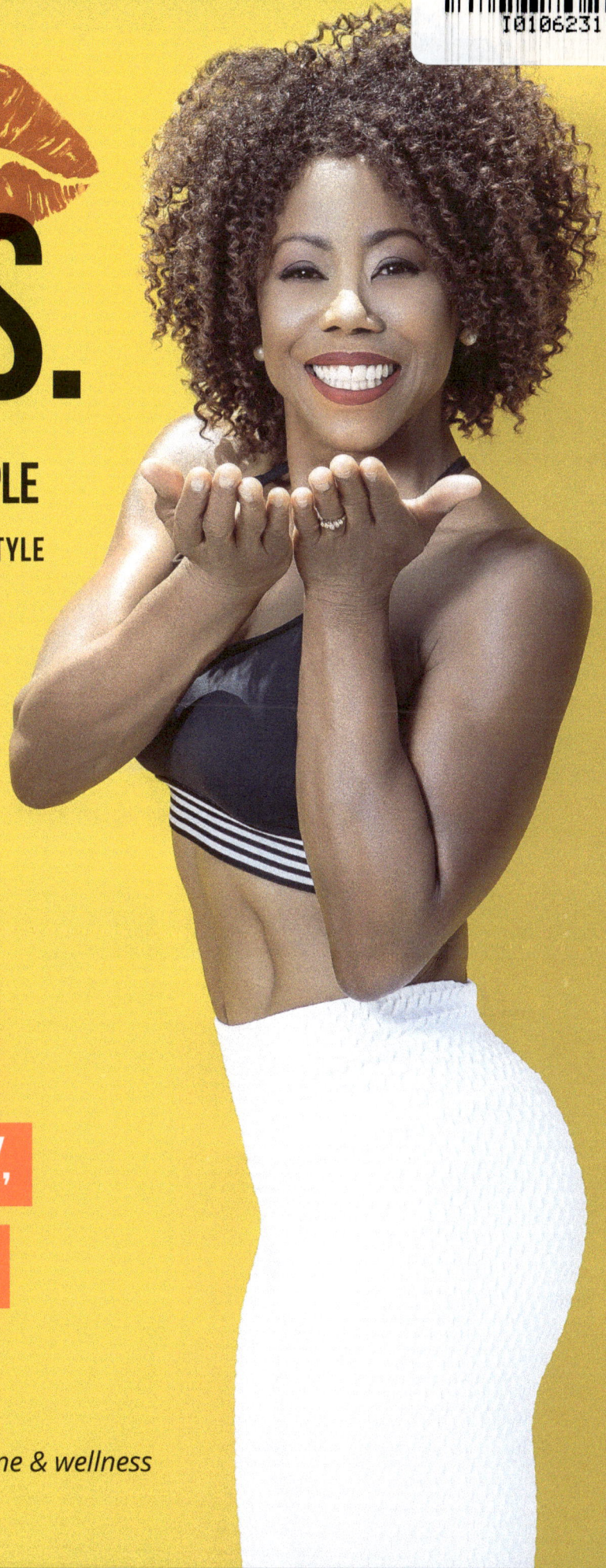

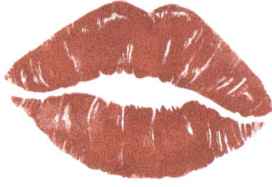

K.I.S.S.:
KEEP IT SHORT AND SIMPLE FOR A HEALTHY, SUSTAINABLE LIFESTYLE,
SECOND EDITION

Cover and book design by João Américo / Book Design by Natalie Minh Interactive

Cover photo & photos on pages 13, 15, 25, 58 (Plank), 59 (Tricep Dips), 75, & 81 © João Américo Fotógrafo

Photos on page 51 © Sami Vaskola

Photos on pages 4, 87 © Perlablue Photography

Photos on pages 3, 17, 18, 58 (Push-Ups), 59 (Lunges & Toe Raises), 60, 70, & 74 © Blue Panda Photography

Photos on pages 11, 85, & 89 © Fitisin Photos/Gordon Smith

Photos on page 92 © Naturalbodybuilding.com Photography

Enchiladas photo on page 65 © Mark Mitchell, https://creativecommons.org/licenses/by/2.0/legalcode, https://www.flickr.com/photos/96741530@N00/6527584289.

Stock images from www.rawpixel.com, www.unsplash.com, and www.pexels.com

"Casper Slide" ("Cha-Cha Slide") written by Marvel Thompson / Willie Perry Jr. / Casper Hudson Beaudy and performed by Willie Perry Jr. Lyrics © Spirit Music Group. All rights reserved.

"Cupid Shuffle" written and performed by Bryson Bernard. Lyrics © The Bicycle Music Company. All rights reserved.

"Electric Slide" written by N. Livingston and performed by Marcia Griffiths. Produced by Island Records. © BMG Rights Management. All rights reserved.

"Wobble" written by Frank Ski, Jonathan Dumas, Jonathan Wright, Michael Crooms, Scott Pajaro, and Victor Owusu. Lyrics © Sony/ATV Music Publishing LLC. All rights reserved.

Printed in the United States of America
ISBN: 978-1-953535-61-0

www.opt2bfit.com | www.trinawiggins.com
Instagram: @trina.r.wigginsmd
Facebook: trina.wiggins.79
Twitter: @trinawiggins123

To those who pursue
daily movement, good nutrition, and peace of mind.

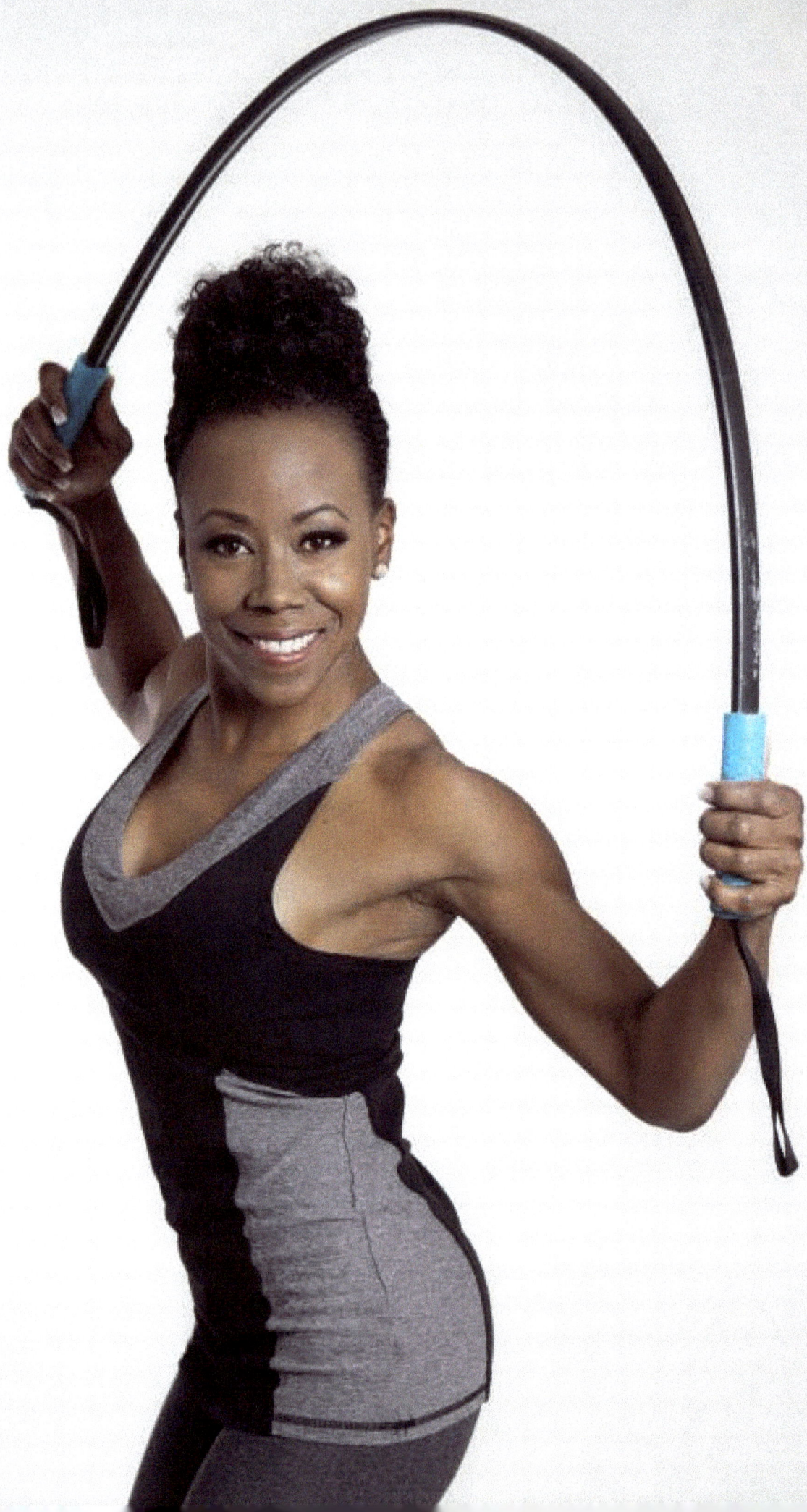

CONTENTS

ACKNOWLEDGMENTS

Being blessed with the opportunity to combine my profession of pediatrics and my passion for fitness to help others navigate a healthy lifestyle has been pure joy. Over the past 32 years, I interacted with family and friends who participated in my journey and helped cultivate my health beliefs. My journey began at the age of 15 when my late father, Curtis Wiggins, was diagnosed with leukemia. At his young age of 35, it was difficult to understand how and why this had happened. My mother began researching and learning all she could about optimizing nutrition for my dad. She began juicing raw vegetables, fruit, and wheatgrass. Unfortunately, my dad was not receptive to the notion of eating plant-based foods to help improve his body's ability to fight disease. Despite his passing away, I learned so much. I decided I wanted to become a physician and learn more about how food impacts health. I am forever grateful to my mother, Barbara Wiggins, whose health vision laid the foundation and planted the seeds of health and nutrition at an early age.

I would also like to personally thank my husband, Dr. Carl Allen, for his unwavering support, encouragement, and love over the years. I want to express a special thank-you to my sister, Tamara Steele, for encouraging me to revitalize my gymnastics skills to compete in fitness shows. I am beyond thankful to my brother, Curtis Lorenzo Wiggins, for his thoughtful, analytical, and editorial assistance every step of the way. My son, Malcolm Allen, also volunteered his time to assist me with editing and proofreading, and for that I am very fortunate and grateful. I am incredibly thankful for my twin sons, Marcus and Malcolm Allen, for not only being honest taste testers for my recipes and smoothies but for also being volunteers at my fitness and nutrition camps. I am also so appreciative of my daughter, Atoya Collins, and my granddaughter, Kellsi Patterson, for being the biggest cheerleaders of my fitness competitions. I want to extend my gratitude to my mother-in-law, Georgia Lee, for also being an honest taste tester of my recipes and, more importantly, for passing along the word of health and nutrition to her family and friends in Mississippi. Last and certainly not least, I sincerely appreciate my fellow Stanford University alumnus, Richard Craven, for always being in my ear and encouraging me to write this book.

"I WANT TO THANK GOD FOR WAKING ME UP IN MY RIGHT STATE OF MIND AND GIVING ME THE ACTIVITY OF MY LIMBS."

—GRANDMOTHER ELDORA

INTRODUCTION

Over the years, I have had a countless number of people ask me, "What's your secret to staying in shape?"

My typical response used to be that it comes down to a healthy diet and workout routine, after which I would share a few examples of foods I ate and exercises I did.

While some people are receptive to this fundamental lifestyle advice, I have noticed that many are intimidated by the mere thought of implementing what they consider an overwhelming change.

I realized I had to find a way to convey my methods for a healthy life in a way that could resonate with anyone, regardless of their previous fitness experience and current work schedule.

Keep It Short and Simple

The most important thing I have learned over the years is this: to get the results you want from any nutrition or exercise program, you must stay consistently consistent.

Progress evolves from a growth mindset and the belief that you can continue to grow and improve. You can cultivate this mindset with a sense of gratitude for where you are and for the small incremental steps along the way. The importance of a grateful mindset cannot be overlooked or discounted.

Like my dear grandmother always said: "I want to thank God for waking me up in my right state of mind and giving me the activity of my limbs."

> ## "YOU WILL NEVER CHANGE YOUR LIFE UNTIL YOU CHANGE SOMETHING YOU DO DAILY."
> —JOHN C. MAXWELL

With this in mind, I decided to take it upon myself to gather all my knowledge and experience—as an athlete, a doctor, and a busy mother of twins, and narrow it down to an easy, understandable guide that everyone can use.

I know all too well how our busy society and the constant pressure to perform can make us feel like there is no time left to take care of ourselves.

This book addresses the issue of self-care in the context of modern demands and constraints.

I have been an athlete for as long as I can remember. Ever since medical school, I tried to figure out how to incorporate fitness into my life. The demands became even greater with my internship and residency, along with being a wife and mother of twins. This situation appeared like the perfect set-up for sacrificing my fitness goals.

Many people get so frustrated and overwhelmed that so-called "paralysis by analysis" strikes. Paralysis by analysis is an inert and unproductive state that prevents people from taking any actionable steps toward achieving their health and fitness goals. However, as stubborn as I am, I refused to let my career and other life commitments compromise my health. I made it a point to incorporate healthy living into my daily routine. Mission accomplished!

Now I want to share with you all the things I have learned along the way so that you can start living a less stressful, more positive, and overall healthier, happier life. By the end of this book, you will realize that it is unnecessary to force yourself to exercise at the end of a long workday or attempt complicated healthy recipes when you are exhausted and uninspired.

This book is about finding lasting balance. It is about implementing one small habit or change at a time and finding smart but simple solutions you can stick to for the rest of your life.

Finally, thank you for making me part of your exciting journey. I sincerely hope that you find my advice not only helpful but also inspirational and motivational. If you ever feel discouraged, just remember that it's not about perfection. The journey to a healthy, sustainable lifestyle is about progress and doing the best you can with what you have.

01

HOW IT ALL BEGAN

Fitness has been a lifelong passionate journey for me and an adventure filled with challenges, victories, and countless revelations. To me, health and wellness are about so much more than just achieving a weight-loss goal or winning a fitness contest. The ideal goal is to live your best life loving your body and thriving in every aspect.

My career as a doctor has taught me that every person is unique and that the definition of optimal fitness, as well as the road to achieving it, is different for everyone. It is about finding that sweet spot where you feel at peace with your life, your body, and your choices. To find it, you must prepare for a journey that may include some trial and error. But remember, some of the world's most incredible scientific discoveries were the result of someone's fearless curiosity and refusal to give up. Everyone has potential waiting to be unraveled and refined. All you need to do is start somewhere.

Now, let me tell you a bit about who I am and where I come from.

MY STORY

One hot summer afternoon, as I was lacing my tennis shoes to play kickball with the kids on 63rd Street in Oakland, California, something caught the corner of my eye. The 1972 Olympics was on TV in the background, and when I looked up, I noticed something that would change the course of my young life. The Russian gymnast, Olga Korbut, was executing a no-hand backflip on the balance beam. Olga was 17 years old, and I was 11 years old at the time.

I remember getting so excited at the sight that I yelled to my mother at the top of my lungs to come see Olga. I was instantly mesmerized and couldn't wait to learn more about this amazing sport.

After watching the Olympic gymnastics events, I looked in the Oakland Yellow Pages to find gymnastic classes. Unfortunately, there were no facilities in Oakland, so I asked my mother to drive me to the Berkeley Public Library to check all the Yellow Pages in the surrounding cities. I checked out 12 phone books on my quest to find a competitive gymnastics club, and finally, I stumbled upon Diablo Gymnastics Club in Walnut Creek, California.

I started with two classes a week. In between classes, I practiced all kinds of flips on my mother's vinyl carpet runner. I quickly progressed, and it did not take long before I moved up from class 3 to class 1.

Upon entering the ninth grade, school and gymnastics became more demanding. As I was now a class 1 gymnast, training was more rigorous and time-consuming.

Thanks to a supportive administration, the academic dean gave me special permission to leave school at 1 p.m. and hop on the Bay Area Rapid Transit (BART) to get to gymnastics practice at 2 p.m.

Practice took place from 2 p.m. to 7 p.m. with a study and food break at 4 p.m. Once practice finished, I would jump back on BART to get home to study. Except for a late dinner pause, I would study from the moment I got home until it was time for bed.

There was no gymnastics practice on Sundays, but as I could not bear to go a day without practicing, I asked my mom for a balance beam so I could continue to perfect certain tricks.

At the tail end of high school, I was planning to participate in tryouts to become an elite gymnast. As I moved up the ladder, my family and I began to notice unusual judging practices. It was during this time when I started to realize the lack of diversity in gymnastics. While competing in the sport, I never saw another Black gymnast other than my younger sister!

One particular incident that stands out the most happened during a competition in Arizona in the mid-1970s. I vividly remember the gymnastics meet was coming to an end, and the judges were beginning to add up the scores. All the gymnasts were eagerly awaiting

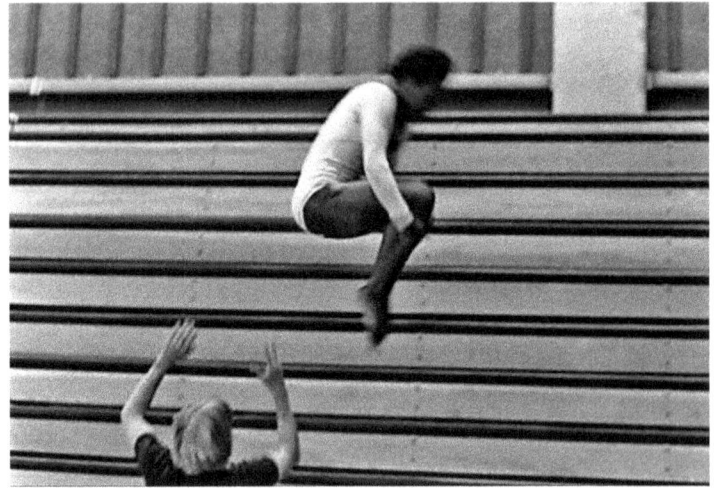

the medal ceremony. After adding up my scores, I came in second place. Right before the awards presentation, the head judge called an immediate judges' meeting. Lo and behold, scores and placings changed, and I found myself in fifth place.

Unfortunately, these unfair judging practices became more and more apparent to me. I quickly realized that I always had to outperform my competitors just to get equal recognition. In other words, I had to be a super gymnast. I simply could not afford to make any mistakes, which amounted to unrealistic pressure for even the most ambitious and passionate young woman.

Therefore, as heartbreaking as it was to defer my dreams of becoming an elite gymnast, I decided to take a break from the sport and focus my energies on getting into college. My life began to shift in a new and exciting direction when I received an acceptance letter from Stanford University.

Upon arriving at Stanford, I made it a point to visit the women's gymnastics coach. I decided to try out for a spot on the team. I remember eagerly waiting to find out if I would become one of the first African American pioneers in women's gymnastics at Stanford University. I couldn't wait to resume training for my floor exercise routine and front tuck vault; they were my favorite events!

ONE WEEK AFTER TRYOUTS, I LEARNED THAT I HAD RECEIVED A SCHOLARSHIP TO STANFORD UNIVERSITY.

Being an athlete and a premed student at the same time was a challenging feat; my life was a constant cycle of study, class, train, eat, sleep, and repeat. Despite the additional workload, I loved being a member of the team. I established longstanding friendships that are still very dear to me.

Sadly, after two years on the team, I sustained an ACL (anterior cruciate ligament) injury to my right knee while competing in Hawaii. I vividly remember the bumpy ambulance ride to the hospital where I received x-rays; my knee would gyrate in pain with even the slightest divot in the road.

I recall having to take a six-hour flight with my leg throbbing in pain. It was excruciating.

Within a week of being back at school, I made the difficult decision not to return to gymnastics. Instead, I chose to focus on healing and applying to medical school.

My four years at Stanford flew by. Suddenly, I was graduating with a BA in human biology and getting ready to head off to Washington University School of Medicine in St. Louis, Missouri. I could not believe I was leaving California for the Midwest!

I pulled into St. Louis on a hot, humid day in mid-August 1982 and set my eyes on the Gateway Arch for the first time. It was breathtaking, and I still remember the feeling of anticipation as if it were yesterday.

I later moved into the medical school dorm where the first person I crossed paths with turned out to be none other than my future husband, Dr. Carl Allen.

Carl had just graduated from Vanderbilt University, and it turned out that he, too, was an athlete. Carl played free safety on Vanderbilt's football team, but just like me, he had sustained an ACL injury to his right knee. The odds of us both having the same scar on the same knee were minuscule, and we laughed plenty at the incredible coincidence.

Carl and I contemplated how we, as former athletes, would be able to work out while in the trenches of medical school. I figuratively remember eating, sleeping, and drinking medical school with virtually no room in my schedule to go to the gym. As a result, practicing time management became an absolute must.

Since I had to do at least some physical activity to stay sane, I invested in a stationary bike. I biked 20 minutes in the morning while reading over my notes. This simple daily routine became etched in stone throughout medical school, my internship, and my residency.

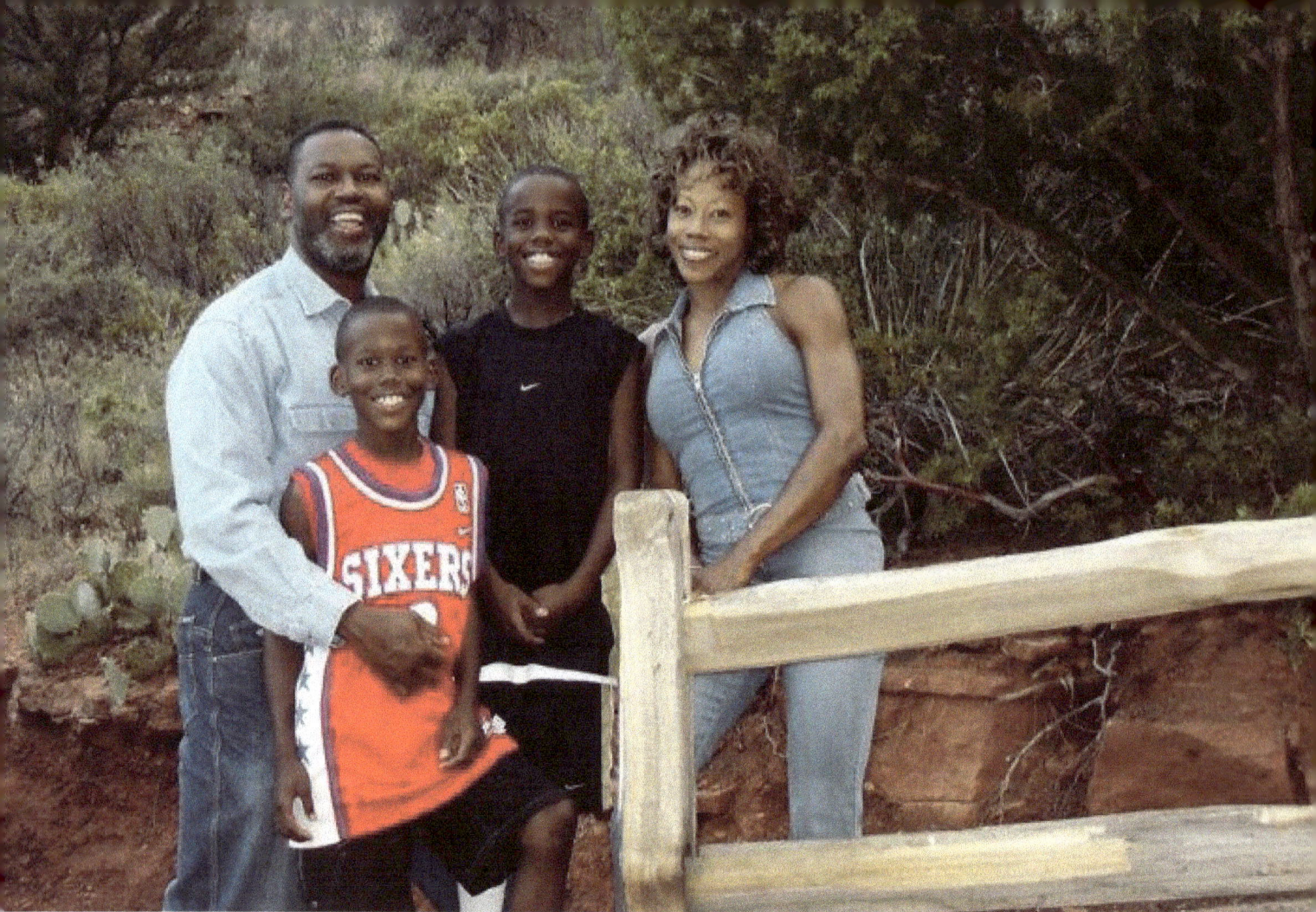

After completing our medical residency programs, Carl and I started our family. My life now included two demanding jobs: full-time pediatrician and mother of twin boys. With my schedule filled to the brim, I did not have the same time for exercise as I did in college. However, being a firm believer that every problem has a solution, I invested in a Stairmaster. I rotated my workouts between the bike and the Stairmaster, maintaining 20 minutes a day.

When the twins were babies, I would put one baby in his infant carrier next to me on the bed and breastfeed the other one while riding the bike. I was burning calories in two ways at once: riding the bike and breastfeeding.

Once the children got a little older, I incorporated more physical fitness activities, like hiking, into my daily routine. The city of Phoenix, where we moved after I completed my residency, boasted spectacular hiking trails, including Squaw Peak and Camelback Mountain. Now with more opportunities for exercise, my husband and I began a joint training routine that included regular power walking in the mountains.

They say couples who work out together stay together, and in that case, we were winning! Not only did we share workouts, but we also shared the challenges of working in the medical field while raising twin boys.

COMPETITIVE FITNESS

While searching for a wedding venue with my sister in 2003, we stumbled upon Ms. Fitness USA at the Rio Resort and Casino in Las Vegas, Nevada. Since the wedding coordinator was running late, my sister suggested that we go and see what it was all about. Much to my surprise and delight, we saw several competitors performing floor exercise routines very similar to those in gymnastics.

It seemed like a perfect fit, and my sister immediately challenged me to participate in these competitions. When I returned home, my mind was spinning. Could I still do the splits, cartwheels, and handstands at the age of 42? After two years of procrastination, I finally put my fears aside and decided to get serious about competition prep.

To get started, I went to my local YMCA and found the tiny tots' cheerleader instructor, who agreed to help me create a gymnastics routine. As I needed to revitalize my dormant skills, I also joined an adult gymnastics class where I could relearn back handsprings and handstands.

For Ms. Fitness USA competitions, the contest requirements included not only performing a floor exercise routine, but also participating in a swimsuit, evening gown, and speech round. Determined to succeed, I began preparing rigorously for all aspects to once again compete at a high level. My goal was to deliver a technically clean and engaging routine along with a meaningful and relevant speech. After listening to many of my competitors' speeches about how fitness had impacted their lives, I decided to take a different approach. I combined my profession of pediatrics with my passion for fitness to address the childhood obesity epidemic. I broadened my discussion of fitness and nutrition with my patients and their families. I made it a point to discuss and distribute my personally designed handouts about tasty, healthy eating and simple ways to exercise. I also expanded outside the office and sponsored fitness and nutrition camps at the Boys and Girls Clubs and local health clubs. I have competed in over 50 shows since 2003, with many top-place finishes. The most notable ones were Triple-A Fitness and Aerobics 11th Legacy International, 2007—1st place; Ms. Fitness USA, 2010—6th place; Ms. Fitness World, 2010—12th place; Fitness America Classic Division, 2011—1st place; Sin City Natural Fitness Championship, 2015—1st place; NaturalBodyBuilding.com Team USA, Grand Masters, 2017—1st place; Nevada Senior Games Dance Category, 2013, 2015, and 2018—Gold Division; and AAU Universe/ICN Las Vegas Fitness International, 2019—1st place.

At this point, I have spent 19 years of my life competing in various fitness, talent, and dance shows. To execute my routine, I have to stay in shape by doing cardio, strength, and flexibility exercises. Performing on stage and entertaining the crowd gives me additional purpose to maintain my physical fitness. It also motivates me to inspire others to be fit. Therefore, I always win, no matter how I place in the competitions. Over my 60 years, I have learned that certain things just work. One of them is that you must keep your exercise routine short and simple, which I refer to as **K.I.S.S.—KEEP IT SHORT AND SIMPLE.**

One of the most common reasons why people fail in their fitness endeavors is because they make things far too complicated. The simpler you make the plan, the more likely you are to stick to it.

Another thing I have learned is that as you get older, you must balance keeping fit with avoiding injury. Stretching and flexibility are important throughout life, but they become increasingly critical as we age.

Finally, you do not have to work out for one continuous hour. Many people never even attempt to get in shape because they erroneously believe spending hours in the gym is the only way to get results. That is simply not true!

You can and will get great results by performing your workout in small chunks throughout the day. And guess what? Your body will not know the difference! Instead of stressing yourself out about fitting one hour of nonstop exercise into your schedule, just devote anywhere between 10 to 20 minutes three times a day. And voila, you have completed a thorough workout without making even the smallest change to your schedule.

Short-interval training is just as effective as a full hour of low-to-moderate intensity training. The golden key is to make it a habit.

— BEING CONSISTENTLY CONSISTENT IS THE KEY!

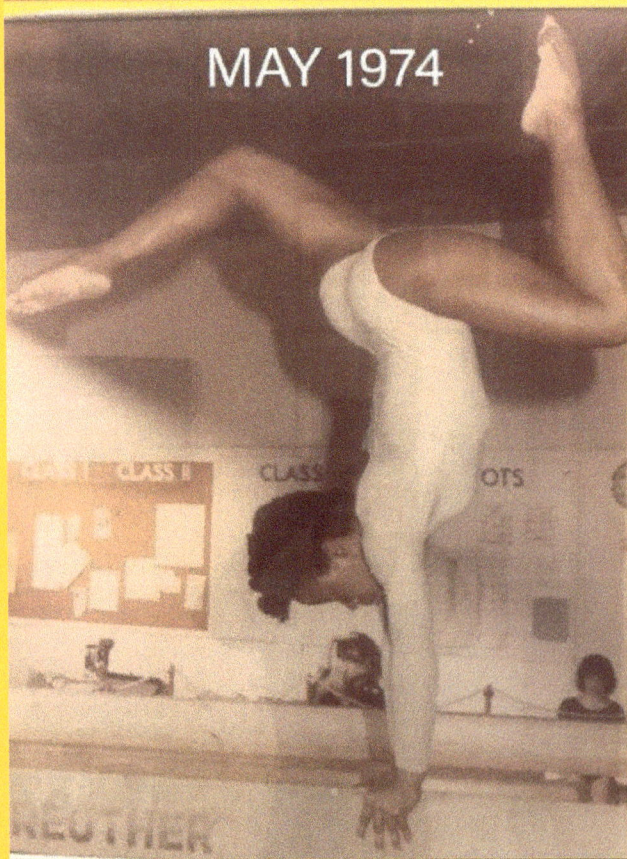

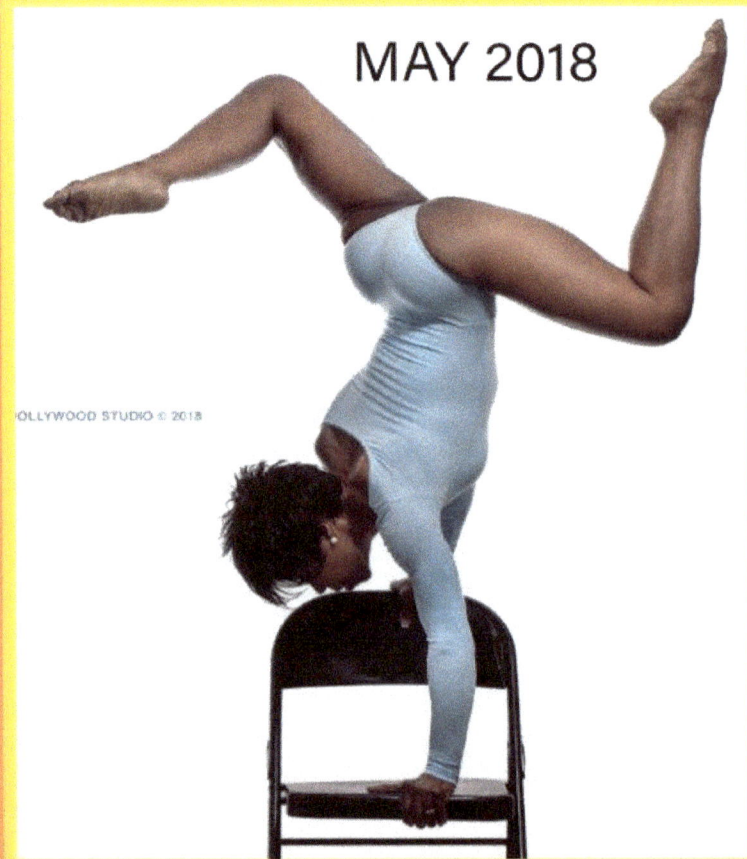

MAY 1974

MAY 2018

> ## "SEEMS IMPOSSIBLE UNTIL IT'S DONE."
>
> —NELSON MANDELA

YOUR NEW LIFE AWAITS

I hope these first few pages have given you a boost of hope, confidence, and encouragement to face the journey ahead.

Fitness can and should be a rewarding and energizing part of your life, not a chore that makes you feel tired and overwhelmed!

I want you to look at this book as your guide that provides the tools, inspiration, and courage to transform your existence little by little, piece by piece. My wish for you is that by demonstrating my approach to everything in life—methodically, patiently, and with the big picture always in the back of my mind—you will learn how to reach your goals with small, actionable steps. Trust me! These steps will take you further than you ever could have imagined.

My approach to fitness is not achieving a fast and temporary transformation.

I believe that the key to attaining lifelong fitness is a combination of patient practice and a steady mind shift toward powerful, healthy habits.

This book is neither a quick fix nor is it a cookie-cutter program that you will toss after a week of boredom and frustration.

It is an informative and practical self-help guide and workbook designed to help you find your way toward feeling physically, nutritionally, and mentally fit.

ARE YOU READY TO TRANSFORM? LET'S GET STARTED!

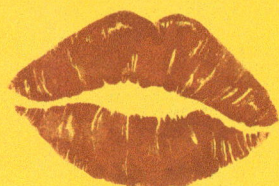

PART 1

DAILY FITNESS ROUTINES

10-20-30 INTERVAL TRAINING

Did you know that smaller intervals of exercise are just as effective as hour-long sessions? Not only are smaller intervals effective, but they can also save you precious time. In our hectic society, time is priceless, and after a long day of hard work, most people do not have the time, will, or energy to spend hours in the gym. Short intervals of exercise with varying degrees of intensity scattered throughout the day are far easier to wrap one's mind around. Therefore, short interval training makes for a more practical and realistic strategy in the long term. Another name for this type of training is HIIT, also known as high-intensity interval training. Don't let the high intensity scare you! It simply means varying your speed up or down during your training.

What are the benefits?

The major benefit of interval training is that you burn more calories. The more intensely you exercise, the more calories you burn, even if it's just for a few minutes. Besides burning more calories, you will enhance your endurance in a fraction of the time and improve your performance and speed. You will also feel less blasé about your workout with the change in levels of intensity. Furthermore, it can be good for your health. A 10-20-30 interval training study done at the University of Copenhagen in Denmark showed improved cardiovascular profiles in trained runners.[1] Their cardiovascular profiles revealed reductions in resting systolic blood pressure and decreases in cholesterol. Hopefully, this study may inspire sedentary individuals to start interval training. In addition to the possible health benefits, consistent interval training at varying levels of intensity scattered throughout the day is not only compatible with a hectic schedule, but it also breaks up the monotony.

Another bonus is that this method is beneficial for all levels and forms of physical fitness. You can choose an appropriate activity that you prefer, whether it be walking, jogging, biking, or climbing stairs.

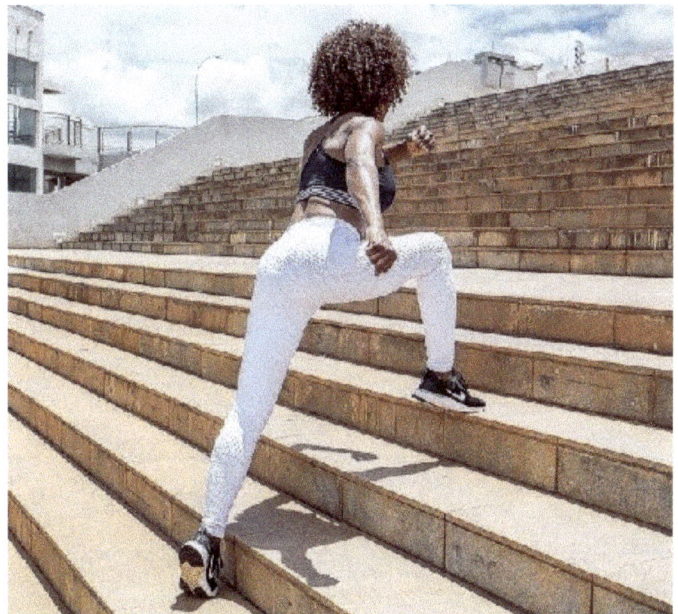

HOW DOES IT WORK?

Choose the activity you wish to do. For 30 seconds, go at a steady, moderate pace (30% of maximal intensity). Then for 20 seconds, pick up the tempo to a moderately fast pace (60% of maximal intensity). Finally, for 10 seconds, go as fast as you can (90% of maximal intensity). You can do this sequence five times with a 2-minute rest and repeat it either immediately or later for a daily total of 30 minutes. The table below shows an example of what this would look like for walking.

— ACTIVITY	— INTENSITY	— DURATION
Walk/Power Walk	30% of max intensity	30 seconds
Jog/Run	60% of max intensity	20 seconds
Run/Sprint	90% of max intensity	10 seconds
		TOTAL: 1 minute = 1 cycle
	Start with 5 cycles, rest for 2 minutes, and repeat if you are able; if not, repeat at a later time to reach 30 minutes a day.	**REPEAT 30 times with a 2-minute rest after 5 cycles**

This workout structure will allow you to achieve better outcomes in half the time. Since a lack of time is the most common excuse for avoiding physical activity, why not try short interval training? I simply walk, jog, or dance for a count of 30, then pick up the pace for a count of 20 and finally give it my all for a count of 10.

The time goes by swiftly with this method. You can easily convince yourself to start and finish the entire workout (even if you do not feel like it) because it consists of small, digestible pieces that add up over time.

NOW THAT WE HAVE GOTTEN TIME OUT OF THE WAY, WHAT IS YOUR EXCUSE?

CASPER SLIDE AND CUPID SHUFFLE

You probably know that the names mentioned above are upbeat songs often played as highlights at weddings or parties. As a fitness competitor, I have learned to incorporate dance into my exercise routines because it brings me joy, happiness, and positive vibes. Research supports the positive effects I experience. The cover article of Stanford Magazine's May 2019 issue, "Why Dance Matters," references a 2003 study in *The New England Journal of Medicine,* and it showed how dancing is beneficial not only for your physical well-being but also for your mental well-being. A large group of senior citizens who danced for five years had a decreased risk of dementia.

So, why not practice your dance moves *and* exercise at the same time?

My tip is to find the extended version of each song and then repeat it until you have reached a total of more than 15 minutes. If you want to step up the intensity, add calisthenics to the dances. For those unfamiliar with calisthenics, they are exercises in which you use your body weight. These exercises involve pushing, pulling, jumping, and running without the use of equipment.

Some examples of calisthenics that you can incorporate into your dance routine include squats, lunges, push-ups, crunches, and jumping jacks. The options are endless!

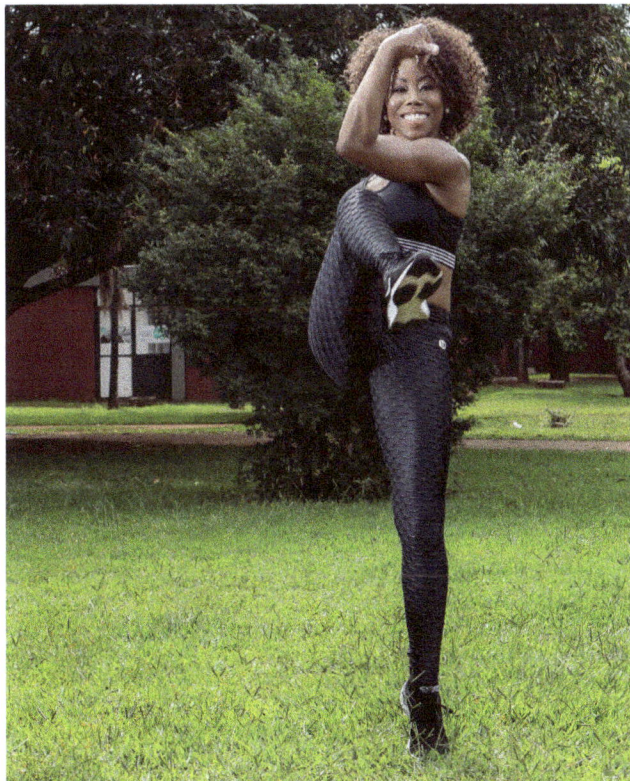

TWISTING CRUNCHES

When I perform the "Casper Slide," I typically add **jumping jacks** when the song says, "One hop this time!"

When the song says, "Stomp!" I incorporate **squats or lunges**.

When the song says, "How low can you go?" I do **push-ups**.

I also work out to the "Cupid Shuffle," and when the song says, "Now kick, now kick!" I do twisting crunches, i.e., opposite knee to elbow.

IT IS JUST LIKE PLAYING SIMON SAYS! CAN YOU IMAGINE A MORE FUN WAY TO GET IN SHAPE?

WORKOUT APP AND OBSTACLE COURSE

We live in an exciting time of evolving technology, so why not take advantage of it? An ever-growing abundance of fitness apps is available these days, many of which will help you get in shape without ever having to step foot in a gym. Since it is just you and your smartphone, nothing is preventing you from getting your workout in regardless of where you are or what you are wearing.

My all-time favorite app is **7 Minute Workout**. This 7-minute model involves 12 high-intensity bodyweight exercises that you perform for 30 seconds each with a 10-second rest in between each exercise. It's an excellent app for anyone who wants to get in a quality workout when time is limited. And beginners will have no problem following along because every exercise includes a short video demonstration on how to perform each movement correctly.

These workouts are both fun and varied with bodyweight exercises like jumping jacks, wall sits, push-ups, abdominal crunches, chair step-ups, squats, tricep dips,

planks, lunges, push-ups and rotations, and side planks.

If you want even more variation, you can always change the exercise and incorporate burpees, mountain climbers, nontraditional push-ups, varied sit-ups with straight legs or bent legs, or walking planks.

7 Minute Workout is the number one fitness app in more than 100 countries because it **keeps exercise short and simple.** (K.I.S.S., remember?) And best of all, it's free!

You can design your very own 7-minute workout using a homemade obstacle course. Create seven stations that include jumping jacks, burpees, mountain climbers, jump rope workouts, agility ladder drills, and step box exercises. Do 1 minute per station or 30 seconds per station twice. You can google specific agility ladder drills, jump rope workouts, and step aerobics routines to incorporate in your obstacle course.

STAIR WORKOUT

Stairs provide the perfect opportunity to incorporate fitness into your everyday life. They are simple tools that are super practical and easily accessible.

In terms of physical benefits, a stair workout will do more than build cardiovascular endurance; it will also improve your lower body, core, and even arm strength.

If you have stairs in your house, you are golden. If you are not so lucky, you can probably find some stairs in the park, in nearby buildings, or in your workplace.

SINGLE-STEP WALKING, JOGGING, RUNNING

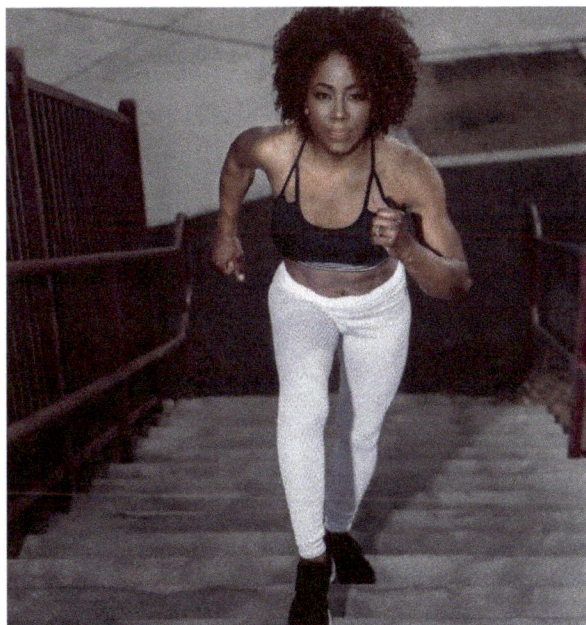

DR. TRINA'S STAIR ROUTINE

The park across the street from my neighborhood has a set of stairs that I use often. I turn on my favorite music and begin my routine, which consists of the following:

SKIP-A-STEP WALKING, JOGGING, RUNNING

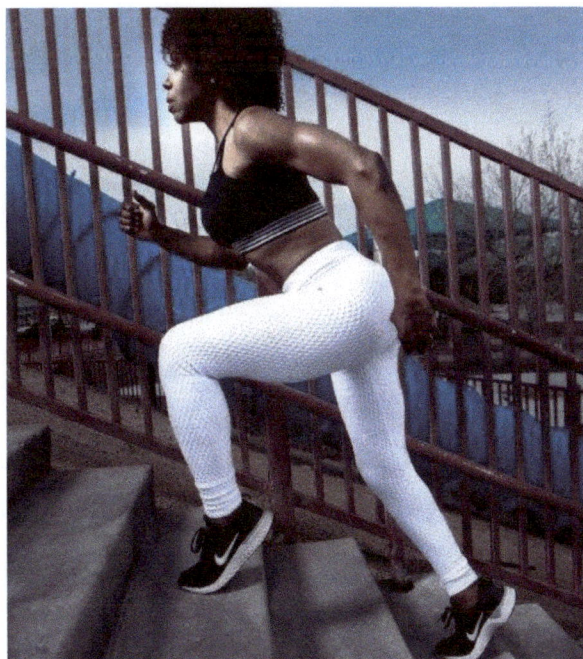

SIDE-STEP CROSSOVER

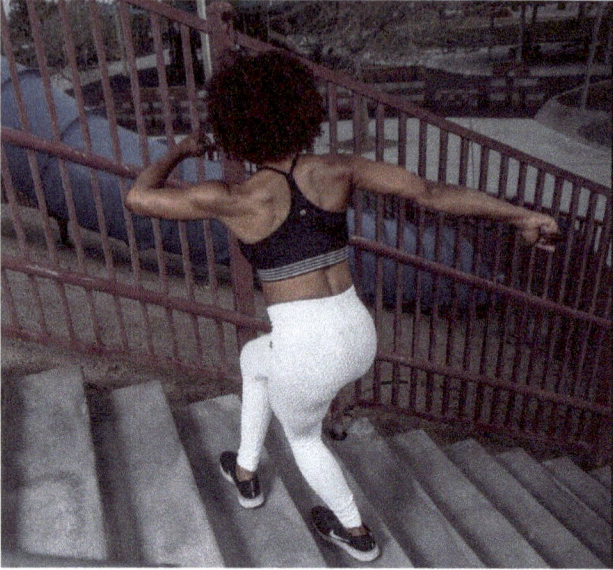

PUSH-UPS ON THE BOTTOM STAIR

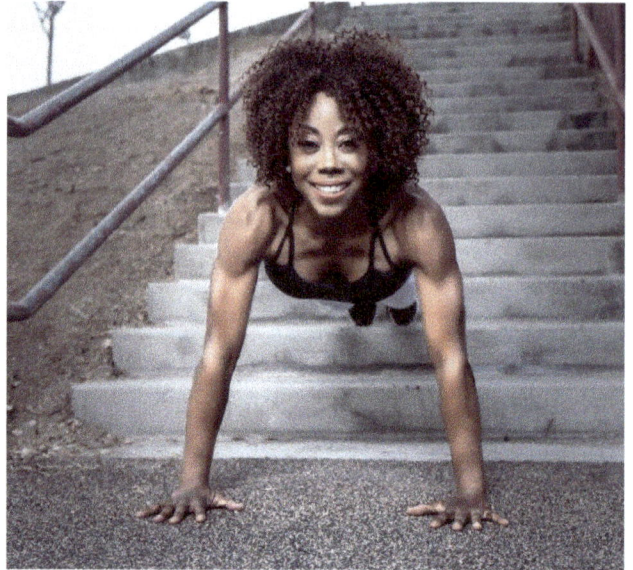

SQUAT JUMPS

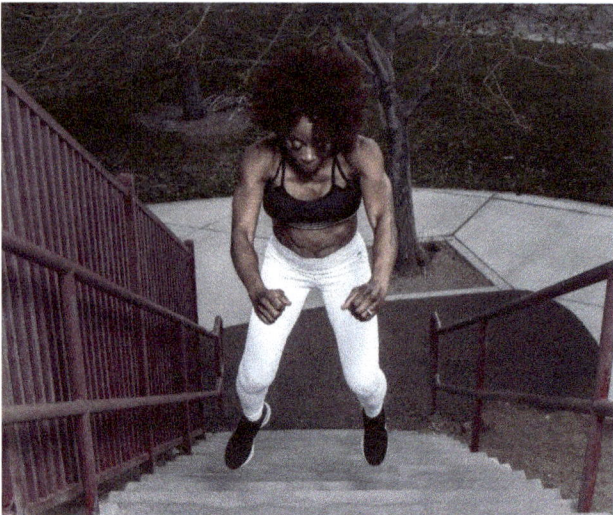

SKIP A STEP WITH ONE LEG WHILE KICKING THE OTHER LEG BACK

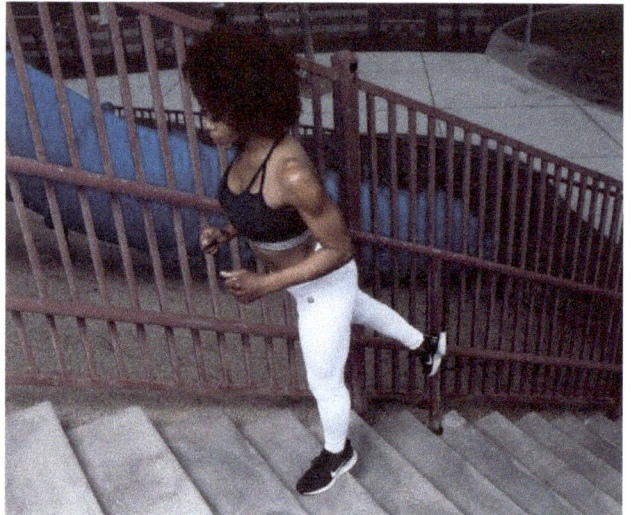

TIPS:

- YOU CAN WALK, JOG, OR RUN DEPENDING ON HOW YOU FEEL THAT PARTICULAR DAY.
- AFTER EACH EXERCISE, JOG OR WALK BACK DOWN THE STAIRS.
- PERFORM EACH EXERCISE THREE TIMES.

N.E.A.T. — NON-EXERCISE ACTIVITY THERMOGENESIS

Non-exercise activity thermogenesis refers to body movement that occurs throughout our daily activities—in other words, unplanned exercise.

To put it simply, N.E.A.T. consists of your daily routine from the time you wake up until the time you go to bed. It is also contingent upon your overall activity level, such as whether your job keeps you moving or sedentary throughout the day.

N.E.A.T. involves finding more ways to activate your body while performing day-to-day activities and incorporating increased movement into your everyday routines.

A great example is to add movement when you take a shower first thing in the morning—an opportunity that most people miss. I always take this chance to stretch my arms, back, and legs. It is incredibly revitalizing, and it gets your day off to a terrific start! Actively seeking opportunities to enhance movement in the moment is akin to practicing mindfulness in the moment as you build body awareness.

Here are other small and simple habits that will help you maintain and build strength and endurance:

- When going to the grocery store, park far from the entrance to gain more steps.

- Use a shopping basket instead of a cart; it forces you to carry your food.

- When you are on the phone, pace around instead of sitting down.

- Always choose the stairs instead of the elevator or escalator.

- When standing in line, do toe raises, toe taps, and shoulder rolls.

- If you are stuck in traffic, do neck rolls and shoulder rolls.

- If you are sitting at the bus stop or subway station, do toe raises, leg extensions, knee raises, arm stretches, side bends, neck rolls, shoulder rolls, wrist circles, ankle circles, or toe taps.

- If you have a desk job, consider using a stability ball or a standing desk.

HOW MANY CALORIES CAN YOU BURN?

The numbers below give you an overall idea of how much energy it takes to perform everyday activities. Now imagine how much more you could burn by incorporating additional movement and increasing your intensity while doing them!

Note: The following examples are guidelines based on a 150-pound person.

CALORIE-BURNING ACTIVITY	15 MIN.	1 HOUR
Sweeping carpets or floors	39	156
Cleaning, heavy or major, vigorous effort—including washing car, washing windows, cleaning garage	34	136
Mopping	43	170
Multiple household tasks all at once, light effort	26	102
Multiple household tasks all at once, moderate effort	43	170
Multiple household tasks all at once, vigorous effort	51	204
Cleaning, house or cabin, general	34	136
Cleaning, light—including dusting, straightening up, changing linen, carrying out trash	26	102
Washing dishes while standing	22	88
Washing dishes and clearing dishes from table with some walking	26	102
Vacuuming	43	170
Cooking or food preparation—including use of manual appliances while standing or sitting	17	68
Serving food, setting table	26	102
Cooking or food preparation with some walking	26	102

Feeding animals	26	102
Putting away groceries, carrying packages—specifically, carrying groceries, shopping without a grocery cart	26	102
Carrying groceries upstairs	111	442
Food shopping with or without a grocery cart, standing or walking	22	88
Non-food shopping, standing or walking	22	88
Ironing	22	88
Sitting—knitting, sewing, light wrapping of presents	9	34
Doing laundry, packing suitcase while standing, folding or hanging clothes, putting clothes in washer or dryer	17	68
Putting away clothes, gathering clothes to pack, putting away laundry while walking around	22	88
Making the bed	17	68
Moving furniture and household items, carrying boxes	85	340
Scrubbing floors on hands and knees—including scrubbing bathroom, bathtub	48	190
Sweeping garage, sidewalk, or outside of house	51	204
Packing/unpacking boxes, light to moderate effort, occasional lifting of household items while standing	43	170
Putting away household items while walking, moderate effort	34	136
Watering plants	26	102
Moving household items upstairs, carrying boxes or furniture	136	544
Light home activities while standing—including pumping gas, changing light bulbs	17	68
Walking, light, non-cleaning—readying to leave, shutting/locking doors, closing windows, etc.	34	136

Activity		
Sitting—playing with child(ren)—light, only active periods	26	102
Standing—playing with child(ren)—light, only active periods	31	122
Walking/running—playing with child(ren)—moderate, only active periods	51	204
Walking/running—playing with child(ren)—vigorous, only active periods	68	272
Carrying small children	34	136
Child care: sitting/kneeling—dressing, bathing, grooming, feeding, occasional lifting of child—light effort, general	26	102
Child care: standing—dressing, bathing, grooming, feeding, occasional lifting of child—light effort	34	136
Elder care, disabled adult, only active periods	51	204
Reclining with baby	9	34
Sitting—playing with animals, light, only active periods	26	102
Standing—playing with animals, light, only active periods	31	122
Walking/running—playing with animals, light, only active periods	31	122
Walking/running—playing with animals, moderate, only active periods	51	204
Walking/running—playing with animals, vigorous, only active periods	68	272
Standing—bathing dog	43	170

DID YOU KNOW?

Did you know that you can calculate how many calories you burn at work by sitting and standing? Go to startstanding.org. Input your gender, age, height, weight, the number of days per week at your job, and the number of hours you spend standing and sitting per day. Then calculate the calories you burn. It is critical to recognize that sitting is the new smoking!

FIND YOUR SPORT

07

"How can I maintain a sustainable workout program? I can't seem to stick to a plan!"

I frequently get this question from people who are frustrated and lost because they keep falling off track despite starting with resolve, motivation, and enthusiasm.

My best tip is simple: find your sport.

If you ever participated in sports when you were younger, whether it was football, gymnastics, or just playing jump rope at school, try remembering how you felt back then. Dig deep and see if you can rekindle that long-lost interest.

For me, performing in fitness competitions and dance shows has given me a purpose to maintain my physical fitness. Performing and regular training are also great ways to clear my mind and escape from our chaotic world. I am confident that most people would benefit substantially from taking up a sport.

Whichever sport you decide upon, it can provide a welcome relief from the daily grind and can also serve as a useful tool to deal with anxiety and stress. Adopting a sport will allow you to refocus your mental and physical energy instead of wasting that energy on nagging worries. Your body and mind will most definitely thank you for this in the long haul.

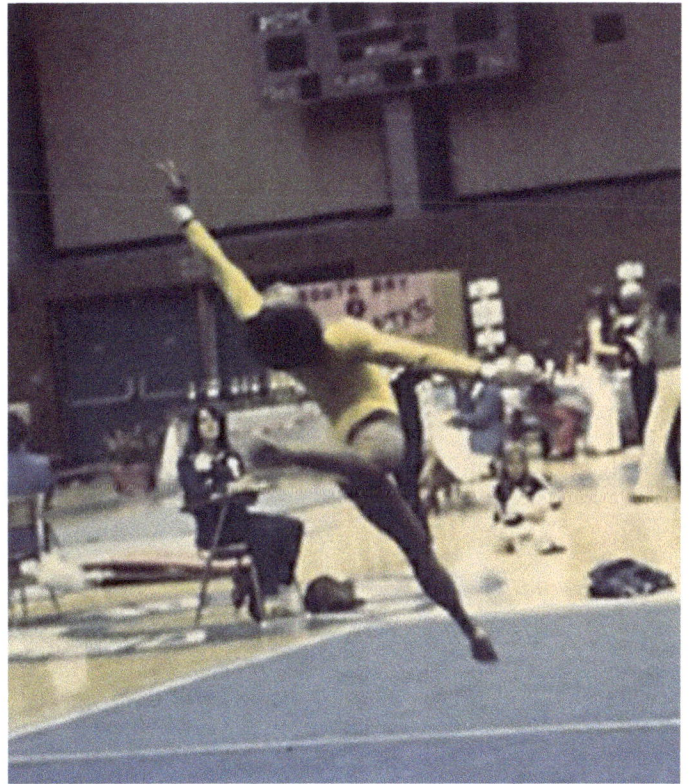

"SPORT SUSPENDS REALITY FOR YOU, ALLOWING YOU A BREATH OF FRESH AIR FROM THE RIGORS OF THE MUNDANE."

—SADHGURU

WHERE DO I START?

Check your local YMCA (1-800-872-9622, www.ymca.net/find-your-y), city recreation centers, and the local or national AAU (Amateur Athletic Union, 1-407-934-7200, https://application. aausports.org/clublocator/) to see if they offer any opportunities for practicing your sport. You should also consider joining an adult league to challenge your mind and body.

If you did not previously participate in a sport, take time to research options that might spark your interest. Once you have decided on an activity, seek out a beginner class and go for it! Remember, the worst thing that can happen is that you do not like it. Even if you don't like it, you will at least be a step closer to finding the activity you do like. Sometimes it takes a bit of trial and error to find "your thing," and that is okay. The trick is to keep trying and never doubt that there is an activity out there that will get you excited and motivated to exercise!

TIPS:

01. Find a physical activity that resonates with you. Make sure it is short, simple, and enjoyable. And remember, exercise is cumulative so integrate it throughout your day. The American Council of Exercise recommends a minimum of 150 minutes of moderate physical activity per week. That equates to 30 minutes 5 days a week. The way you choose to divide your time is totally up to you. My prescription is 10 minutes 3 times a day or 15 minutes twice a day. Dividing the physical activity into small digestible segments scattered throughout the day fosters sustainability. It is so much easier to wrap your mind around short bouts of exercise instead of one long hour session because you can see the light at the end of the tunnel as soon as you begin.

02. To enhance any workout, add 1/2-pound to 1-pound wrist or ankle weights.

03. If you are really pressed for time and are considering not working out, at least do this: **Use the 7 Minute Workout app and perform the one total body stretch as seen on the right for 30 seconds on each side.**

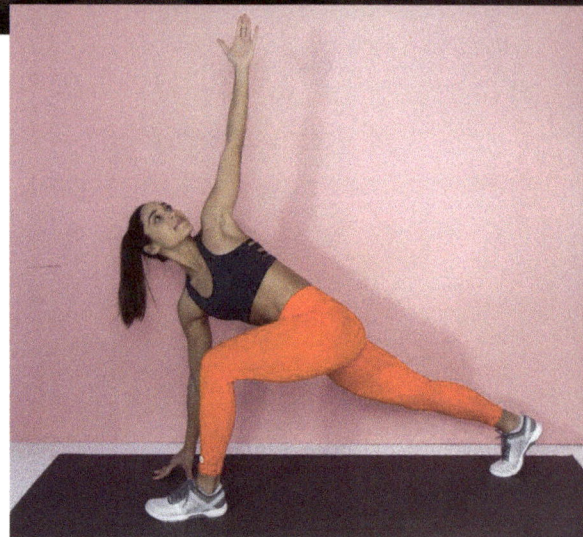

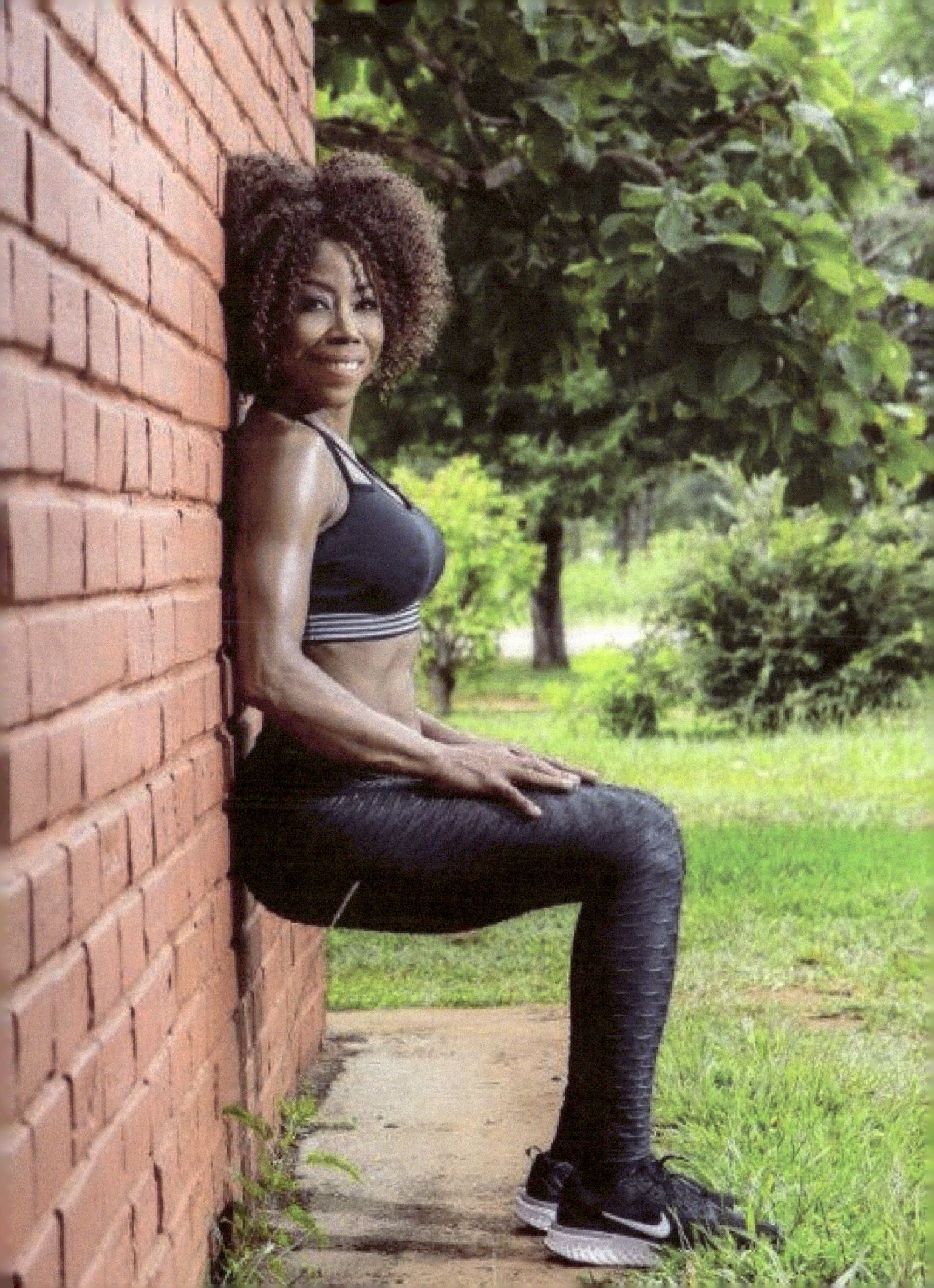

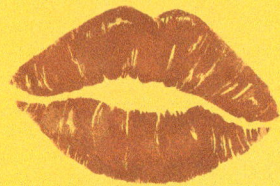

PART 2

MY NUTRITIONAL BELIEFS

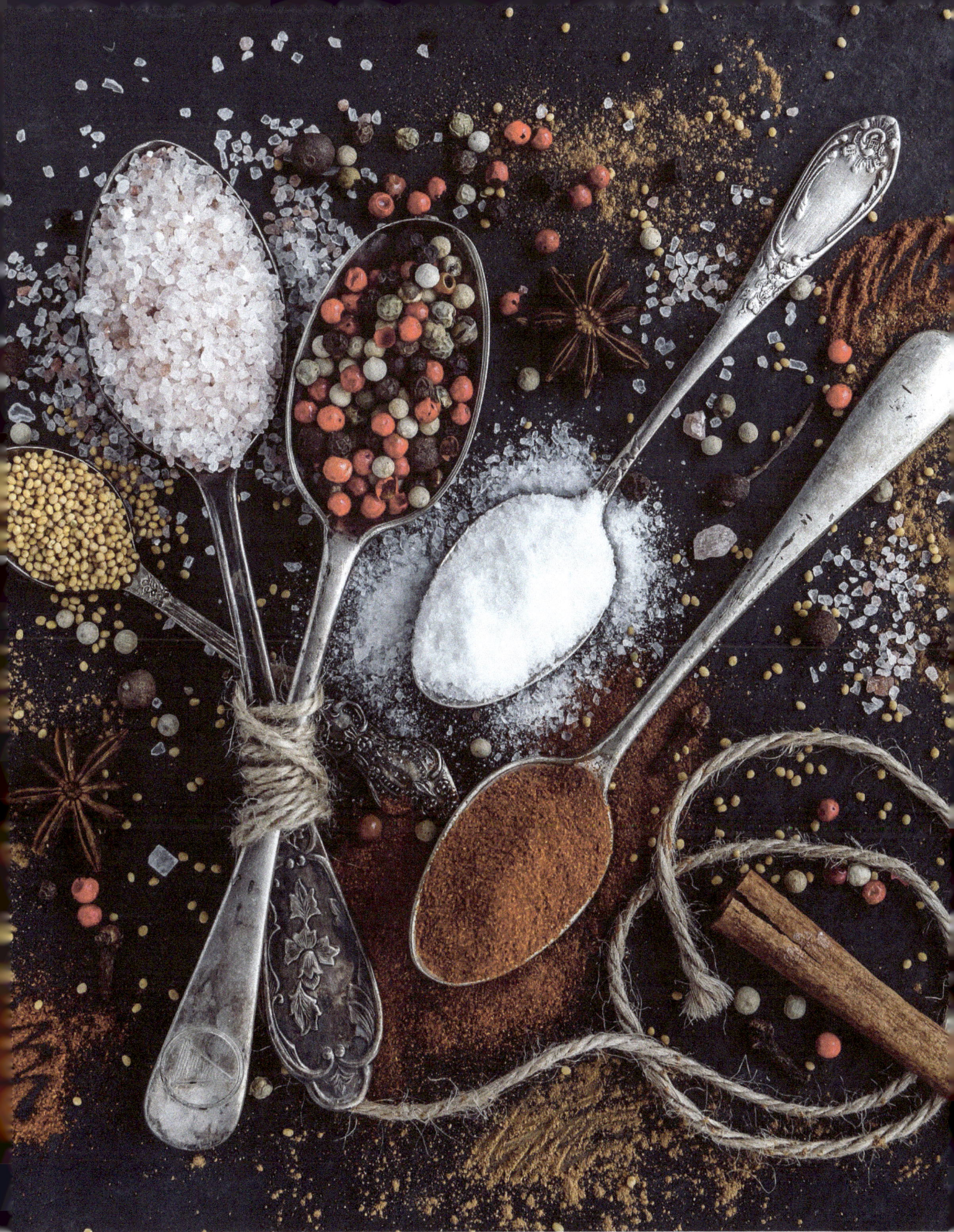

CUT THE SALT

08

Have you ever had swollen feet? Salt could be the culprit since it causes the body to retain water.

Most people have heard at some point that consuming too much salt can lead to hypertension.

We have all eaten a salty meal that made us extremely thirsty. So, exactly how does this happen? Simply stated, water is a magnet to sodium (salt). Wherever sodium goes, water follows. If there is excess sodium within your blood vessels, water will follow, leading to an increased volume of fluid. This increased volume of fluid puts increased pressure on your blood vessel walls. As a result, your blood vessel walls thicken and narrow, thereby creating a smaller opening. Now your heart has to work harder to push blood through narrowed arteries. Subsequently, there is inadequate delivery of blood, oxygen, and nutrients to your body's organs, which can result in heart disease, kidney disease, stroke, and eye damage resulting in blurred vision or even vision loss.

Many people are oblivious to the overabundance of hidden salt in the foods we eat every day!

And guess what? The salt shaker is not the primary offender!

Human beings have used salt as a food preservative for thousands of years, thanks to its ability to prevent spoilage and increase the shelf life of all kinds of food items.

As a result, most prepackaged foods and nearly all restaurant foods today have excessive amounts of salt. It all comes down to profits before health. Without the use of salt to preserve the food, spoilage occurs faster, and food companies ultimately lose money. The Centers for Disease Control and Prevention (CDC) estimates that over 70% of sodium in a typical American diet comes from processed or restaurant foods. Surprisingly, only a small percentage comes from the salt shaker.

Tip: Even though a small portion of dietary salt comes from the salt shaker, it is beneficial to purchase salt-free spices at your local grocery store. Some common brands are Mrs. Dash, Sprouts Farmers Market, The Spice Hunter, and Simply Organic. Use powdered seasoning instead of salts. Refer to the Appendix for a more detailed list.

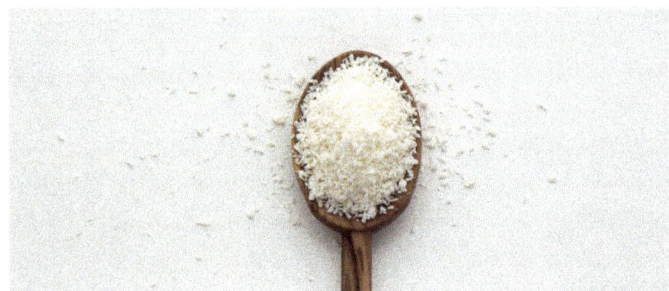

HOW MUCH SALT SHOULD YOU EAT?

The United States Department of Agriculture (USDA) recommends less than 2,300 mg (1 tsp.) of daily dietary sodium.

Ideally, you should aim for no more than 1,500 mg (3/4 tsp.) of salt per day, especially if you are African American, over 50 years old, or suffer from diabetes, hypertension, heart disease, or any other chronic disease. Despite these recommendations, the average American consumes a whopping 3,000 to 6,000 mg of sodium daily.

HOW MUCH SALT ARE YOU ACTUALLY GETTING?

Even if you think your salt intake is low, it can creep up on you unknowingly. To demonstrate, let us look at the sodium (salt) content in a typical sandwich:

- 1 slice of bread, ~200 mg sodium
- 1 tbsp. mayonnaise, ~75 to 100 mg of sodium
- 1 tsp. mustard, ~50 mg of sodium
- 1 slice of American cheese, ~350 mg of sodium
- 2 slices of Oscar Mayer Honey Ham lunch meat, ~560 mg of sodium each

Let's do the math using only the highest of these numbers. If we add together the sodium content from all the listed ingredients, the total salt intake from just one sandwich is **2,020 mg**, a whopping 88% of the recommended daily

amount! Oh, and let's not forget about the chips that often go along with a sandwich. A typical bag of potato chips has about 170 mg of salt per serving.

Remember, this is only one meal. We have not even begun to break down your breakfast, dinner, or, perhaps worst of all, all those snacks!

Now that I have armed you with valuable information regarding the sodium content of a typical American meal, try to be mindful of the things you buy at the grocery store or eat in a restaurant.

If you eat out, look up the nutrition facts first and check the salt content. Many food places now display the full nutrition content of each meal on the menu; however, do not be afraid to ask questions if you cannot locate this information. Your waiter or waitress likely gets a ton of similar inquiries every day!

At the grocery store, make a conscious effort to read the label on all items before purchasing them. Try to limit your purchases of prepackaged foods. Instead, add more fruits and vegetables to your cart. Not only are fruits and vegetables virtually salt-free, but they are also rich in essential vitamins and minerals that your body needs.

Many fruits and vegetables are particularly high in potassium and low in sodium. Our primitive ancestors had a good sodium-to-potassium ratio of 1:16, whereas people today have an estimated ratio of 1:0.7 due to the massive quantities of sodium-laden processed foods. A high sodium diet puts us at an increased risk of hypertension, heart disease, and stroke. So, how can we reverse the ratio?

- Increase potassium-rich foods like apricots, peaches, dates, nectarines, cantaloupes, oranges, figs, bananas, avocados, raisins, zucchini, acorn squash, Brussels sprouts, beet greens, broccoli, collard greens, swiss chard, spinach, and artichokes. Diets high in potassium and low in sodium are associated with a lower blood pressure.

- Limit eating out; many meals are full of sodium. Know the nutritional facts about sodium and other nutrients before you go out to eat.

- Be aware of how much sodium you are consuming daily. Aim for between 1,500 (3/4 tsp.) and 2,300 mg (1 tsp.) per day.

- Decrease your consumption of prepackaged and boxed items.

- Use a variety of salt-free seasoning as well as herbs and spices such as curry, dill, basil, thyme, rosemary, and paprika to enhance the flavor of your meals.

- Minimize the "salty six": breads, cold cuts, cured meats, pizza, poultry, soups, and sandwiches. Make sure you remove the skin on poultry as it is frequently injected with a salt-and-water solution, a process known as brining. Consider cheeseless pizza since many types of cheese contain large quantities of sodium.

- Minimize condiments, frozen foods, canned foods, and pickled foods.

- Try a potassium-rich smoothie: 1/2 cup spinach, 1/2 cup beet greens, 1–2 dates, 1/4 cup frozen peaches, 1/4 cup fresh or frozen pineapple, 1 tbsp. almond nut butter, 1 tbsp. chia seeds, 1/2 cup vanilla almond coconut unsweetened milk, and 1/4 cup crushed ice. Use organic ingredients if possible.

Here are a few examples of common food items and their average sodium content. For a more comprehensive list, visit https://fdc.nal.usda.gov/.

SODIUM CONTENT

DESCRIPTION	MEASURE	SODIUM (MG) PER MEASURE
Thousand Island salad dressing	1 tbsp.	143 mg
Campbell's Chicken Noodle Soup	1 cup	790 mg
Bratwurst—pork, beef, turkey, lite smoked	2.33 oz., one serving	648 mg
Lunch meat—pork, ham, chicken	2 oz., one serving	580 mg
Bagels, plain	one serving	110–418 mg
Tortilla, shelf stable	one serving	364 mg
Canned spinach	one cup	746 mg

CUT THE CHOLESTEROL AND BAD FAT

09

As much as you might love that weekend barbecue, the unfortunate reality is that all meat and all animal-based products contain cholesterol and saturated fat. The FDA tells us that diets high in cholesterol and fat increase the risk of heart disease. New guidelines from the Dietary Guidelines Advisory Committee recommend eating as little dietary cholesterol as possible. For saturated fat, the recommendation is to limit them to less than 10% of the total calories you consume in a day.[1]

"Is cholesterol really that bad?"

Yes, when there is too much of it! Excess cholesterol is the main culprit in causing plaque formation within the arteries, putting you at increased risk for heart disease.

Your liver produces 1 to 2 grams of cholesterol per day to support necessary actions like the production of vitamin D and hormones (estrogen and testosterone). Together, the liver and intestines make roughly 80% of the cholesterol per day to sustain daily bodily functions. For cholesterol to move around the body and perform its job, it needs a transport vehicle. The two most commonly known transporters are HDL and LDL, which stand for high-density lipoprotein and low-density lipoprotein respectively. The good cholesterol is HDL because it picks up cholesterol from the body and delivers it to the liver for removal. On the other hand, LDL is the bad cholesterol because it transports cholesterol to your arteries—a setup for plaque formation and blockage.

In other words, your liver is already doing a great job of sustaining all your vital cholesterol needs. The problem arises when we go beyond the body's natural production and add too much cholesterol to our diet. Excess cholesterol clogs the arteries, leading to heart disease.

Other artery-clogging culprits are saturated fats and trans-fats. Typically, both of these fats are solid at room temperature, like a hard stick of butter. The manufactured form of trans-fat is known as partially hydrogenated oil. Saturated fat comes from animal sources, and trans-fat comes from baked goods and fast foods.

> **TIP:**
> MOST STANDARD GROCERY STORES CARRY MANY PREPACKAGED FOODS THAT CONTAIN PARTIALLY HYDROGENATED OILS, SO MAKE SURE TO CHECK THE LABEL!

Unsaturated fats, on the other hand, are considered good fats. They are considered good for several important reasons, including inducing fullness, assisting in absorbing fat-soluble vitamins (A, D, E, K), composing healthy cell membranes, supporting brain structures, and maintaining healthy skin.

Unsaturated fats consist of two types: polyunsaturated fat and monounsaturated fat. Since these two fats are typically liquid at room temperature, they are not artery-clogging like saturated fats and trans-fats. The most common polyunsaturated fats are omega-3 and omega-6 fatty acids, which are both essential fatty acids. They are 'essential' because our body does not make them. Therefore, we must consume a proper balance of both not only to maintain good health but also to support our heart, joints, brain, mood, and skin. In our society, we eat an abundance of omega-6 and not enough omega-3. Excess omega-6 disrupts the balance between the two, leading to a higher risk of inflammation, a precursor to chronic disease.

Therefore, it's important to consume good sources of omega-3 fats. These include oily fish such as salmon, tuna, herring, mackerel, trout, and sardines. Nuts and seeds are also excellent plant-based sources of omega-3 fats. Conversely, it would be wise to decrease your consumption of omega-6 fatty acids, such as highly refined vegetable oils like corn, canola, cottonseed, soybean, safflower, sesame, and sunflower.

TIP: FAT RECOMMENDATIONS BASED ON THE AMERICAN HEART ASSOCIATION

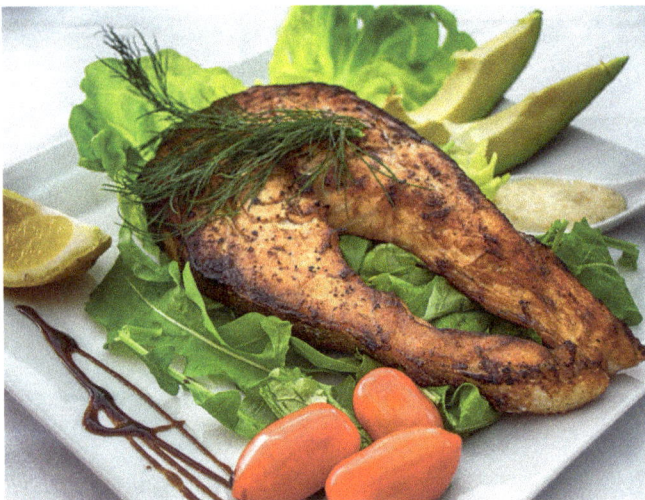

Relish Heart-Friendly Fats: Unsaturated Fats (Polyunsaturated and Monounsaturated) Like Salmon and Avocado

- Decreases your risk of death from heart disease and other fatal diseases
- Decreases your bad cholesterol
- Decreases your triglycerides
- Gives your body the essential fats it needs but can't make

Restrict Heart-Unfriendly Fats: Saturated Fats Like Butter, Cheese, and Salami Deli Meat

- Elevates your risk of heart disease
- Elevates your bad cholesterol

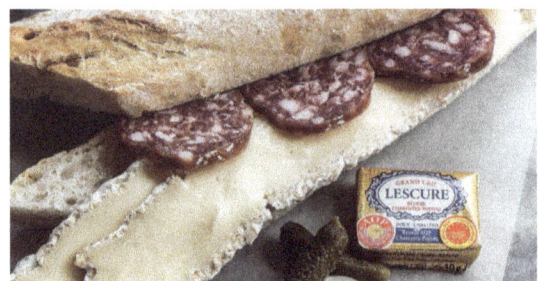

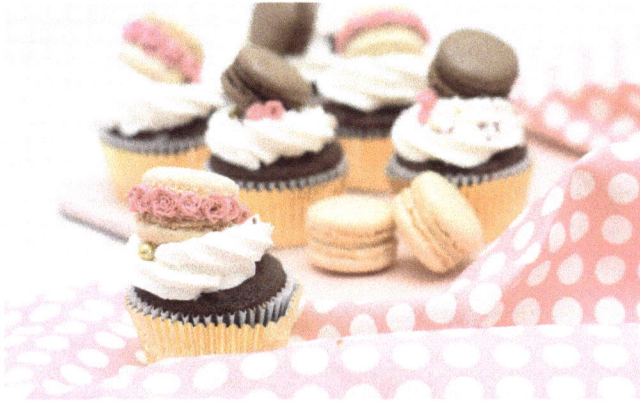

Remove Heart-Unfriendly Fats: Trans-Fats and Hydrogenated Oils Like Desserts Made with Refined, Processed Ingredients

- Elevates your risk of heart disease
- Elevates your bad cholesterol

WHAT ABOUT DAIRY?

Let me put it this way. Can you name any other animal that drinks another animal's milk? Milk and milk byproducts like cheese contain cholesterol and saturated fats, and we have already established they are not good for your heart and arteries. Some dairy products also contain hormones that can disrupt your natural and very delicate endocrine system, thereby creating an imbalance that can cause even more problems.

With there being so many tasty plant-based milk options out there today— almond milk, rice milk, soy milk, hemp milk, cashew milk—why choose cow milk? Besides being tasty, there is less chance for spoilage and waste because plant-based milk does not require refrigeration until after it's opened.

In addition to the variety of plant-based milk on the market, there are several vegetables high in calcium, including spinach, kale, okra, and collard greens. Other foods high in calcium are white beans, soybeans, sardines, salmon, perch, and rainbow trout. As you can see, cutting back on milk doesn't have to mean sacrificing nutrients.

CONTROLLING YOUR CHOLESTEROL INTAKE

To control how much cholesterol you eat, I recommend you incorporate meatless days throughout the week and reduce your portion size. As a general guideline, the portion size for meat should be slightly less than the area of the palm of your hand. I also suggest that food from plant sources make up the majority of your plate. Small changes over time are the best approach to achieving a healthy diet. Consider starting with Meatless Mondays for one month, then progress to two meatless days per week the following month, and so forth. You can also cut your portion size of meat in half and amp up the number of vegetables and whole grains. Another option is replacing meat with a piece of omega-rich wild-caught salmon or tuna.

THE SECRET TO SERVING SIZE IS IN YOUR HAND

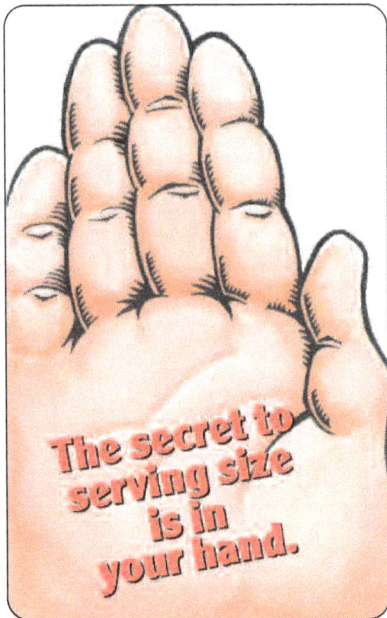

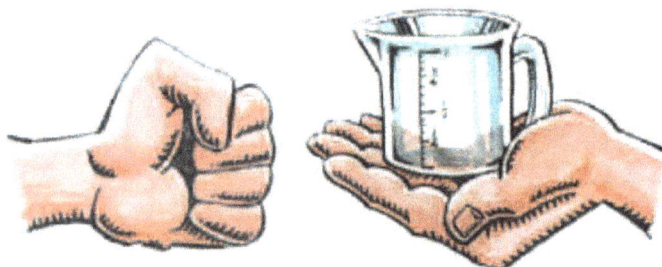

The secret to serving size is in your hand.

A fist or cupped hand = 1 cup

1 serving = 1/2 cup cereal, cooked pasta or rice
or 1 cup of raw, leafy green vegetables
or 1/2 cup of cooked or raw, chopped vegetables or fruit

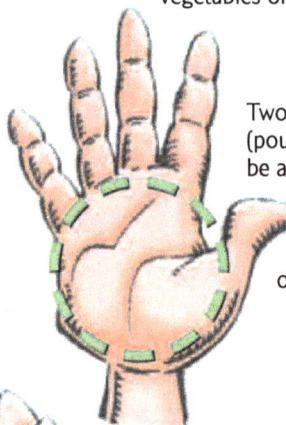

Palm = 3 oz.of meat

Two servings, or 6 oz., of lean meat (poultry, fish, shellfish, beef) should be a part of a daily diet. Measure the right amount with your palm. One palm size portion equals 3 oz., or one serving.

A thumb = 1 oz. of cheese

Consuming low-fat cheese is a good way to help you meet the required servings from the milk, yogurt and cheese group.
1 1/2 - 2 oz. of low-fat cheese counts as 1 of the 2-3 daily recommended servings.

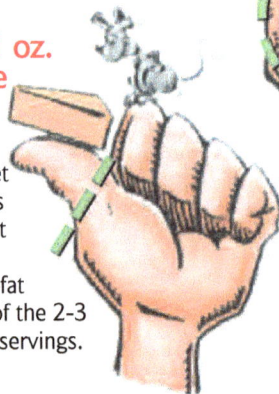

Thumb tip = 1 teaspoon

Keep high-fat foods, such as peanut butter and mayonnaise, at a minimum by measuring the serving with your thumb. One teaspoon is equal to the end of your thumb, from the knuckle up.

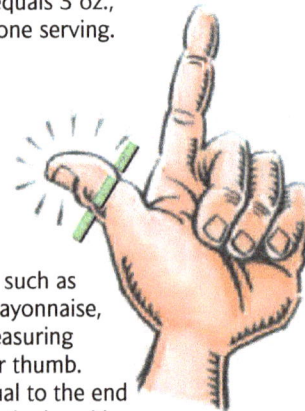

Three teaspoons equals 1 tablespoon.

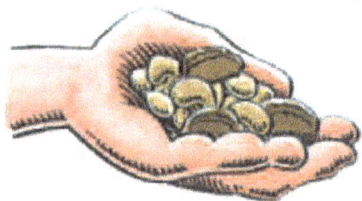

Handful = 1-2 oz.of snack food

Snacking can add up. Remember, 1 handful equals 1 oz. of nuts and small candies. For chips and pretzels, 2 handfuls equals 1 oz.

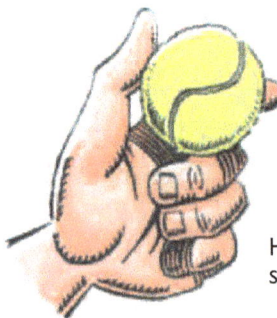

1 tennis ball = 1 serving of fruit

Healthy diets include 2-4 servings of fruit a day.

Because hand sizes vary, compare your fist size to an actual measuring cup.

Color Me Healthy

WHY PLANT-BASED?

There are many benefits to following a mostly plant-based diet.

The International Agency for Research on Cancer, a division of the World Health Organization, has classified processed meats—such as hot dogs, ham, bacon, sausage, chorizo, and deli meat (pastrami, corned beef, salami, and bologna)—as Group 1 carcinogens. Group 1 carcinogens are cancer-causing agents, and these processed meats are no different from alcohol, cigarettes, and asbestos. Furthermore, many studies corroborate these findings and link these meats with an increased risk of colorectal cancer.[1] In addition to processed meats, red meat—such as beef, lamb, and pork—has been labeled as a Group 2A carcinogen, which means there is a strong possibility it causes cancer.

In recent years, there have been plenty of stories in which people radically improved their health by reducing or eliminating animal products from their diet.

One such example is the former president of the American College of Cardiologists, Dr. Kim Williams, who saw his cholesterol and lipid lab profile numbers drop significantly after adopting a plant-based diet. Not surprisingly, Dr. Williams now advises his patients to do the same.

Another example is Seventh-Day Adventists, who promote a vegetarian diet. They have a 30% lower risk of cancer and a longer life expectancy. On average, Seventh-Day Adventist members live about a decade longer than most Americans, and this is primarily due to their plant-based diet, regular physical activity, and avoidance of smoking and alcohol.

I recommend you start eliminating both red and processed types of meats. Twenty years ago, I began my food journey with the elimination of these meats.

My diet subsequently consisted of baked (skinless) chicken and baked, omega-rich fish such as salmon, tuna, and halibut. I do not recommend charring meat because the interaction between meat and high heat produces carcinogenic agents. I eventually eliminated all cholesterol sources from my diet, including chicken, fish, and dairy products. It is important to note that you do not have to be entirely plant-based to get the benefits of reducing your intake of animal products. The key to achieving a healthy body is to make the majority of your plate plant-based and to remove processed meat and red meat.

CUT THE SUGAR

It may taste heavenly, but sugar is one of the most inflammatory and addictive substances you can put into your body. It only takes one bite of sugar to stimulate the brain to release dopamine, a chemical that drives our cravings. Dopamine is the same chemical that causes alcoholics and drug addicts to seek a high again and again. In 2013, a study done at Connecticut College found that in lab rats, Oreo cookies were not only as addictive as cocaine, but they were also more pleasurable. After removing the sugar, the rats experienced teeth chattering, head shakes, and forepaw tremors similar to cocaine withdrawal symptoms. In addition to its addictive nature, sugar has a multitude of other negative effects. Too much sugar can increase your risk of heart disease, type 2 diabetes, kidney disease, cancer, weakened immunity, non-alcoholic fatty liver disease, rheumatoid arthritis, worsening joint pain, obesity, impotence, and depression. It can even accelerate the aging process, causing poor dentition and increased wrinkling and sagging of the skin.

Similar to our discussion in Chapter 8 about hidden salt in our food, there are hidden sugars as well. And believe it or not, all sugar ain't sweet. Many foods are high in sugar but aren't sweet, such as breakfast cereals, salad dressings, sauces, and soups. It is also important to be aware of sneaky sugar aliases on food labels. Other names for sugar include corn sweetener, agave nectar, beet sugar, brown rice syrup, dehydrated cane juice, maltodextrin, malt syrup, sorghum, fruit juice concentrates, high fructose corn syrup, invert sugar, molasses, dextrose, fructose, glucose, lactose, maltose, sucralose, and sucrose.

Moreover, too much sugar causes massive spikes in blood glucose levels and puts an undue load on the pancreas to produce insulin, which may increase your risk of type 2 diabetes. Besides, type 2 diabetes comes with a laundry list of its own problems, such as heart disease, kidney disease, nerve damage, eye disease, and stroke.

Sugar comes from carbohydrates. All of the food we eat breaks down into carbohydrates, proteins, or fats. These three nutrients are also known as macronutrients (see the Appendix for a detailed explanation). Carbohydrates come in two forms: simple and complex. Complex carbohydrates, derived primarily from plants, consist of starches and fiber. Simple carbohydrates and starches both break down into glucose to provide fuel and energy for our bodies. Simple carbohydrates are in many processed foods: white bread, white pasta, white flour, white sugar, brown sugar, candy, soda, syrup, yogurt, fruit drinks, pastries, and baked goods. They are quickly broken down by our bodies, resulting in blood sugar spikes. On the other hand, complex carbohydrates take more time to break down, thereby leading to fewer blood sugar fluctuations. They are typically high in fiber, and foods high in fiber slow down the digestive process. Good sources of complex carbohydrates include 100% whole grains, 100% whole wheat flour, 100% whole wheat bread, oats (rolled or steel-cut), sweet potatoes, yams, lentils, legumes, beans, quinoa, asparagus, green beans, Brussels sprouts, cauliflower, and broccoli.

How do we determine which foods are culprits?

Back in the early 1980s, Dr. David Jenkins pioneered the concept of the glycemic index in his research to determine the best foods for people with diabetes. He analyzed various foods to find out how quickly each food converted to sugar. Each food was subsequently assigned a number from 0 to 100. If the food converted to sugar quickly, a higher number was assigned. If the food converted to sugar more slowly, a lower number was assigned.

The American Diabetes Association and the medical industry generally agree with the numerical ranking of blood sugar known as the glycemic index. Glycemic index values of 55 or less are considered low and deemed good, whereas values between 56–69 are considered moderate and tolerable. Values greater than 70 are considered high and unfavorable.

Knowing the glycemic index is only part of the equation. After establishing the glycemic index, you can also determine the glycemic load, which will give you a more reliable picture. The glycemic load predicts the amount of food required to increase one's blood glucose two hours after eating, depending on the amount of carbohydrates consumed.

If you do a little research, you will find a substantial amount of sugar in many of the foods we eat. Some of the main offenders in our modern society are soda, sugary drinks, candy, and baked goods such as breads, pies, and pastries. You can find a chart of common foods and their glycemic index values at https://universityhealthnews.com/daily/nutrition/glycemic-index-chart. You can also calculate your glycemic load at https://glycemicloadcalculator.com.

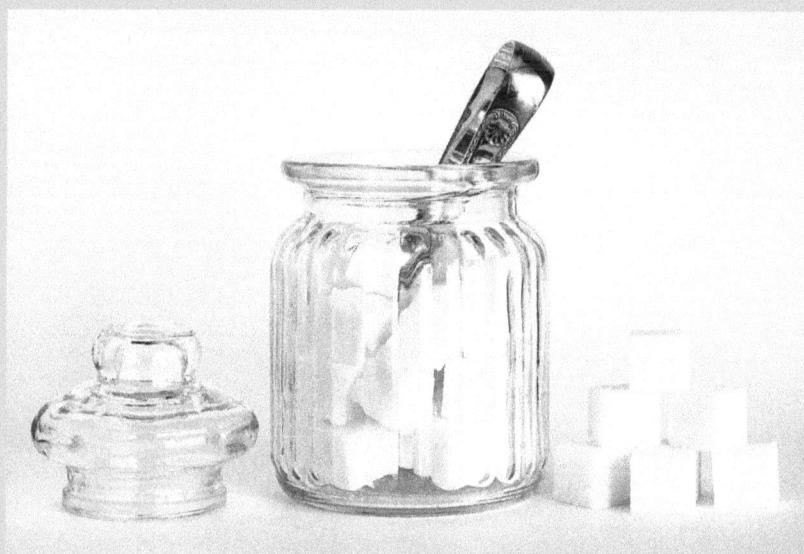

Did you know the average American consumes 19 tsp. (77 grams) of sugar per day? According to the American Heart Association, the maximum amount of sugar per day that a man should consume is 9 tsp. or 36 grams. On the other hand, the maximum amount of sugar per day that a woman should consume is 6 tsp. or 24 grams. (Note: 1 tsp. of sugar equals 4 grams of sugar.)

Trust me, filling that quota goes by much faster than you think! To give you a frame of reference, one 12 fluid ounce can of Coke has 39 grams of sugar, which exceeds the daily allotment for both men and women.

Just one daily can of soda amounts to a staggering 32 pounds of sugar a year. This daily habit will result in a weight gain of at least 15–25 pounds since excess sugar not used to generate energy converts to adipose tissue, also known as fat.

Do yourself a favor and drop the detrimental soda habit. Instead, create your very own soft drink! Mix 1/4 cup of your favorite 100% juice with 3/4 cup of sparkling water. This combination will provide you with much less sugar and no artificial flavors, but plenty of fizz!

As for baked goods, try to limit your consumption without depriving yourself.

My favorite weekly treat is a vegan blueberry muffin or a vegan chocolate chip cookie from Whole Foods.

CUT THE EMPTY CALORIES— ALCOHOL

CHAPTER 11

If you are eating healthy and still not losing weight, the culprit might be those extra glasses of wine or beer. Alcoholic drinks are high in empty calories and have no nutritional value, making it easy to gain weight from drinking too much alcohol.

For example, one bottle of white wine contains approximately 550–600 calories, about 1/3 of the daily calorie intake for women and 1/5 of the daily calorie intake for men.

Treating yourself to two 5-oz glasses of white wine at the end of each day may seem like a harmless pleasure, but those two tiny glasses will provide you with approximately 1,540–1,680 extra calories per week, causing you to gain almost 1/2 pound. Should you keep up this habit, you will add a shocking 24 pounds to your frame in only one year!

When you look at these numbers, it is easy to understand why drinking alcohol is counterproductive to your fitness goals. Besides potentially causing weight gain, too much alcohol taxes your liver and prevents it from performing its duties properly.

An overworked liver may not be able to clear out toxins, ensure a balanced hormonal output, produce adequate amounts of bile, or control sugar and cholesterol levels in your blood. If you compromise these vital functions for any length of time, your body's delicate equilibrium will suffer, and you may experience weight gain and a host of other health issues.

Furthermore, research points to alcohol as the direct cause of certain cancers and an indirect cause of many other cancers.[1] In 2018, a study in *The Lancet Journal* reported that any level of alcohol consumption, regardless of the amount, leads to a loss of healthy life.[2] The study concluded there is no safe level of alcohol consumption.

However, some researchers believe that an occasional glass of red wine may have some health benefits due to an ingredient called resveratrol. These benefits include reducing inflammation, limiting the spread of cancer, lowering cholesterol, lowering blood pressure, protecting brain function, slowing cognitive decline, and easing joint pain associated with arthritis.

To help monitor your alcohol intake, check out one of my favorite online resources, drinkaware.co.uk.

CUT THE PROCESSED FOOD

12

Processed foods are foods that humans have intentionally altered from their natural state. This deliberate alteration of food is a surefire recipe for trouble. Common processed foods include breakfast cereals, breads, cakes, microwaveable meals, savory snacks, white rice, white flour, buns, rolls, canned fruit, canned vegetables, jellies, jams, deli meats, and cured meats.

If you don't want to give up meats, at least remove processed meats (hot dogs, ham, sausage, chorizo, pastrami, corned beef, salami, and bologna). Studies have linked all of these items to an increased risk of colorectal cancer. For a more extensive list of processed foods, please go to nutritiontribune.com.

> **"THE PROBLEM WITH HIGHLY PROCESSED FOODS IS, THEY ARE USUALLY LOADED WITH SODIUM FOR SHELF STABILIZATION, SUGAR FOR TASTE, OR ADDED FATS, INCLUDING SATURATED AND TRANS-FATS, FOR MOUTH FEEL."**
>
> —KRISTI KING, MPH, RDN / REGISTERED DIETITIAN NUTRITIONIST & SENIOR PEDIATRIC DIETITIAN AT TEXAS CHILDREN'S HOSPITAL AND SPOKESPERSON FOR THE ACADEMY OF NUTRITION AND DIETETICS AND KIDS EAT RIGHT

Research has linked highly processed foods to many chronic conditions, including obesity, heart disease, diabetes, and some types of cancer. [1][2][3]

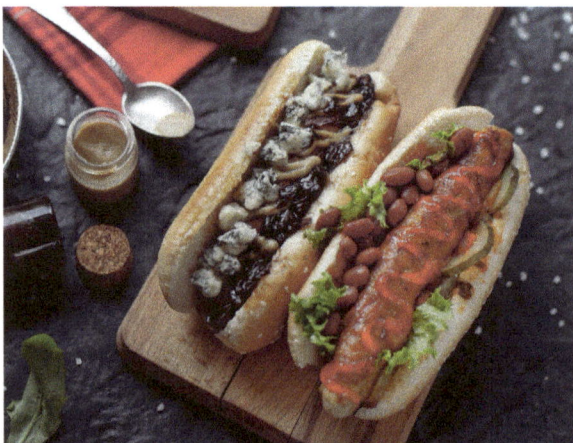

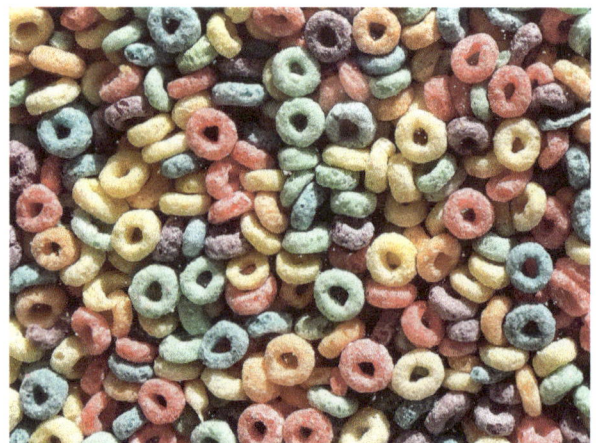

SO HOW DO WE AVOID FALLING IN THE SWAMP OF PROCESSED FOODS?

Increase Your Greens

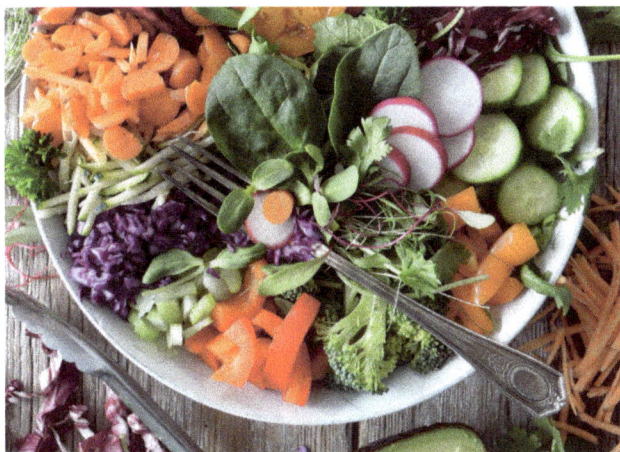

Increasing the amount of greens in your diet is a great way to improve your intake of healthy nutrients and fiber. Implementing this simple nutritional habit will help keep your blood sugar stable and prevent you from craving processed foods.

As for myself, I drink a green vegetable and fruit smoothie most mornings, and I diversify the fruits and vegetables that I use in my meals. You should always try to add greens to your plate. Consider eating a dark, leafy green salad along with vegetables and fruits at lunch and dinner!

Choose Slow Carbs / Complex Carbs

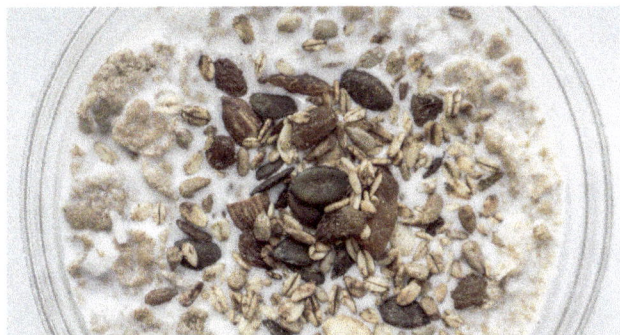

What are slow carbs (aka complex carbs)? Slow carbs take more time to break down in your body, thereby leading to a more gradual release of energy. As a result, you are less likely to see spikes in your blood sugar.

Focus on eating slow carbs such as 100% whole grains, rolled or steel-cut oatmeal, sweet potatoes, yams, lentils, legumes, beans, quinoa, and non-starchy vegetables such as asparagus, green beans, Brussels sprouts, cauliflower, and broccoli. Avoid simple carbs like white bread, white pasta, candy, soda, and baked goods. In general, slow carbs have a lower glycemic index, whereas simple carbs have a higher glycemic index.

Check out www.diabetes.org for a more extensive list of glycemic index foods. Other valuable websites include www.glycemicedge.com, www.verywellfit.com, or www.health.harvard.edu.

Pick Healthier Snacks

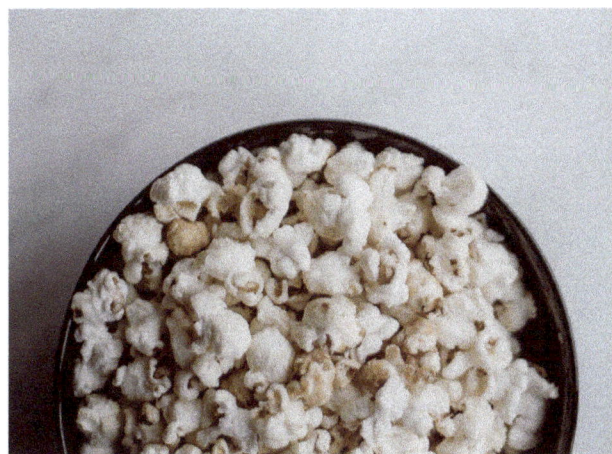

Try sprinkling nutritional yeast on nonfat popcorn. Nutritional yeast has a cheesy flavor, and it's a good source of vitamin B12.

Eat at Home

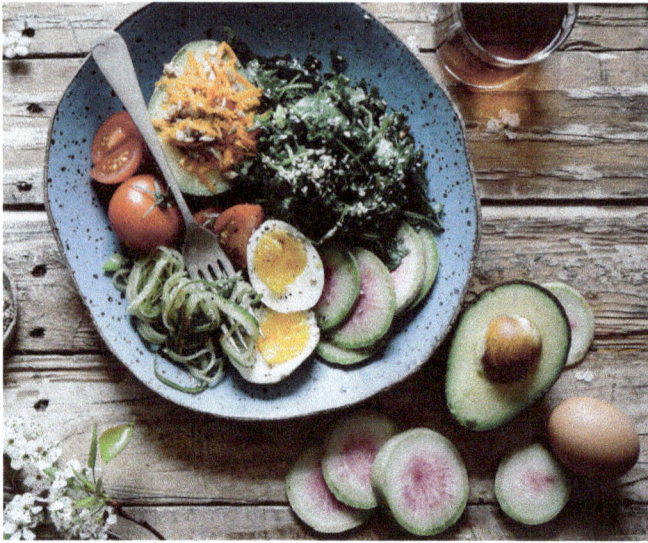

Eat more home-cooked meals and limit the number of times you eat out. Most restaurant menu items contain processed foods with excess salt, sugar, and fat. Eating at home gives you more control over what is in your food and saves you a lot of money in the process—a win-win situation!

Prep Your Meals

Failing to plan is one of the most common reasons why people fall short of eating healthily. Life can be stressful, and there will undoubtedly be situations when you have neither the time nor the energy to stand in front of the stove and cook. It will then be very tempting to reach for prepackaged foods or to head to the nearest fast-food restaurant. On such occasions, having your freezer stocked with precooked, wholesome meals is priceless! I recommend that you pick one or two days during the weekend (or whenever you have time off) to prepare meals for the entire week. It may seem hard at first, but prepping your meals will become second nature once you get into the habit. Doing this will make your life so much easier and healthier in the long haul.

TIPS:

01. If your budget allows, consider hiring a professional chef who is trained in healthy nutrition to show you how to prepare your meals.

02. I recommend getting the book *Eat This, Not That!* by David Zinczenko and Matt Goulding.

03. If I'm in a place with minimal healthy options and my healthy dining app, HappyCow, has no wholesome suggestions, I will look for Chipotle or Panera Bread. These restaurants are in most states.

04. Consider trying meal kits from various companies such as Blue Apron, Home Chef, HelloFresh, Sun Basket, Freshly, or Plated.

FOOD LABELS 101

13

If you are not in the habit of reading food labels or have a hard time understanding them, this chapter will be a serious game changer!

It is important to remember that food companies are predominately interested in getting to your wallet and are less interested in keeping you healthy. As a result, their product marketing is often very deceiving. Buzz phrases like "gluten-free," "fat-free," and "sugar-free" can trick you into believing that you are purchasing a healthy product when you are just buying into the food companies' clever marketing strategy. Something can be sugar-free, gluten-free, dairy-free, or fat-free and still be on the list of unhealthy and highly processed foods. Many food companies simply replace the missing ingredient with another potentially harmful substitute. A great example is companies that remove sugar and replace it with aspartame.

I recommend minimizing the consumption of foods that come packed in a box, carton, or can. These are more likely to be over-processed and have excess sugar and salt. Fresh produce is always your best bet when it comes to clean nutrition—so try to ensure fresh produce makes up the majority of your grocery list.

If you must purchase prepackaged foods, always scan the label for the following items to make sure the product is acceptable.

- Look at the ingredient list first. Do not purchase the food item if the list is long. If you do not recognize the name of the ingredient and can't pronounce the name, then it is probably not suitable to eat.

- Avoid products containing the following ingredients: partially hydrogenated oils, high-fructose corn syrup, sodium benzoate, potassium benzoate, BHA (butylated hydroxyanisole), sodium nitrates, sodium nitrites, MSG, sweeteners, preservatives, artificial flavors, and artificial food coloring.

- Artificial food colorings have possible links to everything from cancer to behavioral issues.

BLUE #1 (BRILLIANT BLUE)
Products to watch out for include: baked goods, dessert powders such as boxed gelatins and puddings, candy items, various beverages, breakfast cereals, and pharmaceuticals.

BLUE #2 (INDIGO BLUE)

Products to watch out for include:
colored beverages, candy items, pet food, and pharmaceuticals.

CITRUS RED #2

Products to watch out for include:
skins of Florida oranges.

GREEN #3 (FAST GREEN)

Products to watch out for include:
pharmaceuticals, personal care products, and certain cosmetic products.

RED #3 (ERYTHROSINE)

Products to watch out for include:
sausage casings, oral medications, maraschino cherries, baked goods, and candy items.

RED #40 (ALLURA RED)

Products to watch out for include:
various beverages, pastries and other baked goods, dessert powders, candy items, breakfast cereals, pharmaceuticals, and cosmetics.

YELLOW #5 (TARTRAZINE)

Products to watch out for include:
pet foods, pastries and other baked goods, various beverages, dessert powders, candy items, breakfast cereals, gelatin desserts, pharmaceuticals, and cosmetics.

YELLOW #6

Products to watch out for include:
colored baked goods, breakfast cereals, various beverages, dessert powders, candy items, gelatin desserts, sausage, pharmaceuticals, and cosmetics.

- Check the serving size and servings per container. Serving size stands for one serving, and servings per container are the total number of servings in the container. When reading the nutritional facts, you must realize that if you eat the entire container of food, you must multiply all the nutrient values on the label by the servings per container.

- Check the calorie content. In general, 40 calories are considered low, and 400 calories are considered high. Calories from fat should be less than 1/3 of the total calories.

- Make sure total fat, saturated fat, cholesterol, sugar, and sodium are as low as possible, and check that these nutrients' %DRV (daily recommended value) is less than or equal to 10%. Ideally, you should aim for zero trans-fat and cholesterol. Eating too much fat, saturated fat, trans-fat, cholesterol, sodium, and sugar will increase your risk of heart disease, high blood pressure, diabetes, and some cancers.

Sample label for
Macaroni & Cheese

① **Start Here** ➡

Nutrition Facts

Serving Size 1 cup (228g)
Servings Per Container 2

Amount Per Serving

Calories 250   Calories from Fat 110

② **Check Calories**

	% Daily Value*
Total Fat 12g	18%
Saturated Fat 3g	15%
Trans Fat 3g	
Cholesterol 30mg	10%
Sodium 470mg	20%
Total Carbohydrate 31g	10%
Dietary Fiber 0g	0%
Sugars 5g	
Protein 5g	

③ **Limit these Nutrients**

Vitamin A	4%
Vitamin C	2%
Calcium	20%
Iron	4%

④ **Get Enough of these Nutrients**

* Percent Daily Values are based on a 2,000 calorie diet. Your Daily Values may be higher or lower depending on your calorie needs.

		Calories	2,000	2,500
Total Fat	Less than		65g	80g
Sat Fat	Less than		20g	25g
Cholesterol	Less than		300mg	300mg
Sodium	Less than		2,400mg	2,400mg
Total Carbohydrate			300g	375g
Dietary Fiber			25g	30g

⑤ **Footnote**

⑥ **Quick Guide to % DV**

- 5% or less is Low
- 20% or more is High

- Look for a high content of dietary fiber, vitamin A, vitamin C, calcium, and iron. With these items, you want the %DRV (daily recommended value) to be above 10%. Remember, fiber is your friend because it binds cholesterol, keeps the colon healthy, helps control weight, removes carcinogenic agents from the body, and prevents constipation.

- Based on the dietary guidelines for Americans, the recommended daily intake for fiber is 14 grams per 1,000 calories. With every 14 grams of fiber consumed, the calorie intake is decreased by 10% because fiber helps keep you full and satisfied.

- Good sources of fiber include fruits, vegetables, and whole grains. A good serving of fiber is around 5 grams. For a man and a woman, the average daily requirement of fiber is 38 grams and 25 grams, respectively.

Nutrition Facts

About 16 servings per container
Serving size 1/4 cup (36g)

Amount per serving
Calories 140

	% Daily Value*
Total Fat 2g	3%
Saturated Fat 0g	0%
Trans Fat 0g	
Cholesterol 0mg	0%
Sodium 0mg	0%
Total Carbohydrate 26g	9%
Dietary Fiber 3g	11%
Total Sugars 0g	
Includes 0g Added Sugars	0%
Protein 4g	
Vitamin D 0mcg	0%
Calcium 9mg	0%
Iron 1mg	6%
Potassium 130mg	2%

GOOD LABEL

Nutrition Facts

36 Servings Per Container
Serving Size 76g

Amount Per Serving
Calories 330

	Daily Value % *
Total Fat 31g	48%
Saturated Fat 11g	55%
Trans Fat 0g	
Cholesterol 65mg	22%
Sodium 1010mg	42%
Total Carbohydrate 1g	0%
Dietary Fiber 0g	0%
Total Sugars 1g	
Includes Added Sugars	%
Protein 13g	0%
Vitamin D	%
Calcium mg	4%
Iron mg	4%
Potassium mg	6%

BAD LABEL

TIP:

THE EASIEST WAY TO REMEMBER THESE DIETARY TIPS IS WHAT I CALL "THE RULE OF 10'S." AT THE VERY LEAST, YOU SHOULD ASCERTAIN THAT THE FAT, SALT, SUGAR, AND CHOLESTEROL ARE EACH BELOW 10 % OF THE DRV (DAILY RECOMMENDED VALUE). ALSO, CHECK THAT THE FIBER AND VITAMINS ARE ALL ABOVE 10% OF THE DRV.

Want to learn more?

I recommend reading *The Safe Shopper's Bible* by David Steinman and Samuel Epstein.

ORGANIC VS. NON-ORGANIC

14

The word "organic" is associated with healthy foods and has been for many years. But what does organic mean?

According to California Certified Organic Farmers (CCOF), organic produce is food grown without using harmful pesticides, GMOs (genetically modified organisms), ionizing radiation, synthetic fertilizers, or sewage sludge. For a product to be marked USDA organic or certified organic, at least 95% of ingredients must be organic, with the remaining percentage consisting of nonagricultural substances that appear on the NOP (National Organic Program) List of Allowed and Prohibited Substances.

If a farmer wants to label his vegetables as organic, he must be able to certify that his produce was grown on soil that had no prohibited substances applied to it for at least three years before the latest harvest.

For meat, poultry, eggs, and dairy products to qualify as organic, the animals must have eaten 100% organic foods throughout their lifetime. They also cannot have received treatment with antibiotics or growth hormones at any time.

Furthermore, organic regulations require that livestock owners raise their animals in conditions that accommodate their natural behaviors; for example, cows should graze on green pasture.

PROCESSED FOOD RULES

Since processed foods contain a combination of ingredients, the rules are slightly different. The USDA organic standards require that these sorts of products contain no artificial preservatives, colors, or flavors. All contents must be organic. There is, however, a minor exception to the latter rule. The USDA does allow processed organic foods to include some approved nonagricultural ingredients, such as enzymes in yogurt or baking soda in bread.

What about companies that state on the package that the product consists of certain organic ingredients or food groups?

A company can technically make this claim as long as the product contains at least 70% organically produced ingredients. The creation of the remaining non-organic ingredients must not have involved any forbidden procedures (for example, genetic engineering).

Although these types of products will not boast the USDA organic seal on the package, they must list the USDA-accredited certifier to verify that the organic ingredient or food group meets USDA's organic standards.

WHAT ARE THE BENEFITS OF EATING ORGANIC PRODUCE?

IMPROVING YOUR HEALTH

Eating organic produce will markedly decrease your exposure to toxic pesticides such as fungicides, herbicides, and insecticides. In conventional produce, the residue from these pesticides remains on the food. Ingesting these pesticides can have negative health implications. Some research has shown that pesticide exposure increases the risk of leukemia, lymphoma, breast cancer, and prostate cancer.[1] Children with developing immune systems are especially vulnerable to toxic substances; therefore, children run an increased risk of developing diseases from such exposures. In addition to the harmful effect of pesticides, a study in *The British Journal of Nutrition* found that organic milk and meat contained a more favorable composition of healthy omega-3s. The author's rationale is that this results from animals foraging on grasses rich in omega-3s instead of being fed an unnatural diet consisting of grains and corn.[2][3] Another significant study included data from a compilation of more than 300 studies demonstrating that organic crops contain notably higher concentrations of various antioxidants as well as potential anti-inflammatory and cell-protective compounds.[4]

HELPING THE ENVIRONMENT

Organic farming is beneficial for our environment because it decreases pollution and enriches both the soil and our ecosystem.

One of the most detrimental effects of producing non-organic or traditional produce is evident in the global decline of the honey bee population. Honey bees are incredibly important to humans; they are the leading pollinator of food crops. If honey bees disappear, it could result in a food supply disaster. There is an association between the decline of the honey bees and pesticide use in industrial agriculture.[5]

EATING ORGANIC ON A BUDGET

Organic foods are typically more expensive and can be a financial burden for many people. One way to circumvent the extra cost of organic fruits and vegetables is to buy organic produce only if the pesticide level is high for a particular fruit or vegetable. In other words, you can purchase conventional produce if the pesticide level is low. (Refer to the following page for the levels of pesticides in different types of fruits and vegetables.)

If you can afford it, choose organic food whenever possible. If you have a choice between prepackaged organic soup and conventional spinach, the better choice by far is the spinach. Just be sure to wash any conventional produce thoroughly before eating it.

To identify a product as organic, check the PLU code (Price Look-Up code). All organic produce has a PLU code that begins with the number 9, while the conventional produce has a PLU code that begins with either a 3 or 4. A PLU code that begins with the number 8 is genetically modified.

The following foods often contain high levels of pesticides:

- Apples
- Bell peppers
- Cucumbers
- Celery
- Potatoes
- Grapes
- Cherry tomatoes
- Kale
- Collard greens
- Squash
- Nectarines
- Peaches
- Spinach
- Strawberries
- Hot peppers

The following foods typically contain low levels of pesticides:

- Asparagus
- Avocados
- Mushrooms
- Cabbage
- Sweet corn
- Eggplant
- Kiwis
- Mango
- Onions
- Papaya
- Pineapple
- Sweet peas
- Sweet potatoes
- Grapefruit
- Cantaloupe

SUPERFOODS

15

While staying active and regularly exercising is critical in terms of physical fitness, none of it will matter if you supply your body with poor nutrition.

Think of your body as an army comprised of billions of soldiers (cells) working 24/7 to keep you healthy and capable of fighting off disease. For this army to fight a good fight and win the battle, you need to arm its soldiers with the right ammunition. In other words, you must give your cells the fuel that they need to thrive.

I have said it before, and I will say it again: the best defense comes from the earth and is not man-made. Earth food includes fruits and vegetables in the produce section of your grocery store.

Fruits and vegetables contain phytochemicals, compounds that give fruits and vegetables their rich, vibrant colors. Berries like blueberries and raspberries are abundant with phytochemicals, as are vegetables such as red beets, spinach, and various colored peppers (red, yellow, and green).

So-called superfoods are the most phytochemical-rich plant-based foods available. These include dark green vegetables, seeds (flaxseed and chia seeds), berries, legumes, oranges, and whole grains.

Consuming plenty of phytochemical-rich foods on a daily basis arms your cells with the best possible ammunition to put up a strong defense against disease and various toxic influences.

HOW TO GET YOUR GREENS IN

Adults need a minimum of five cups of green produce daily to receive basic health benefits. However, nothing is preventing you from exceeding those minimum recommendations. Like I always say, the more, the better!

Some people find it challenging to fill their daily quota of greens. I suggest starting every day with a delicious vegetable and fruit smoothie. This smoothie is the best way to start your day because it ensures that your body gets a wide range of nutrients. Any additional greens from there on will be a bonus.

Try to also fit in a colorful salad with lunch, and add a combination of vegetables, beans, and nuts to your dinner plate. At the very least, make it a rule to eat one form of vegetable with each meal!

Make sure to purchase a variety of vegetables, fruits, and berries since each kind contains a different set of phytochemicals to help build your defense. You can include a plethora of delicious fruits and vegetables to make your smoothie, such as bok choy, kale, spinach, parsley, mangos, pineapples, dates, and all kinds of berries. These are just a few of the many nutrient-rich options that are available in most grocery stores!

DR. TRINA'S GREEN SUPER SMOOTHIE

Makes 1 large serving

INGREDIENTS*

- 1/2–3/4 cup unsweetened vanilla almond coconut milk
- 1/2 cup kale
- 1/2 cup spinach
- 1/4 cup pineapple chunks
- 1 or 2 pitted dates
- 1/2 banana
- 1/8 cup pumpkin seeds
- 1 tbsp. chia seeds
- 1/2 thumb-size turmeric root, peeled or 1/2 tsp. ground turmeric
- 1/2 thumb-size ginger root, peeled or 1/2 tsp. ground ginger
- 1/4 to 1/2 cup frozen blueberries
- 1 tbsp. Sprouts Unsalted Unsweetened Creamy Almond Butter
- 1/8–1/4 cup crushed ice

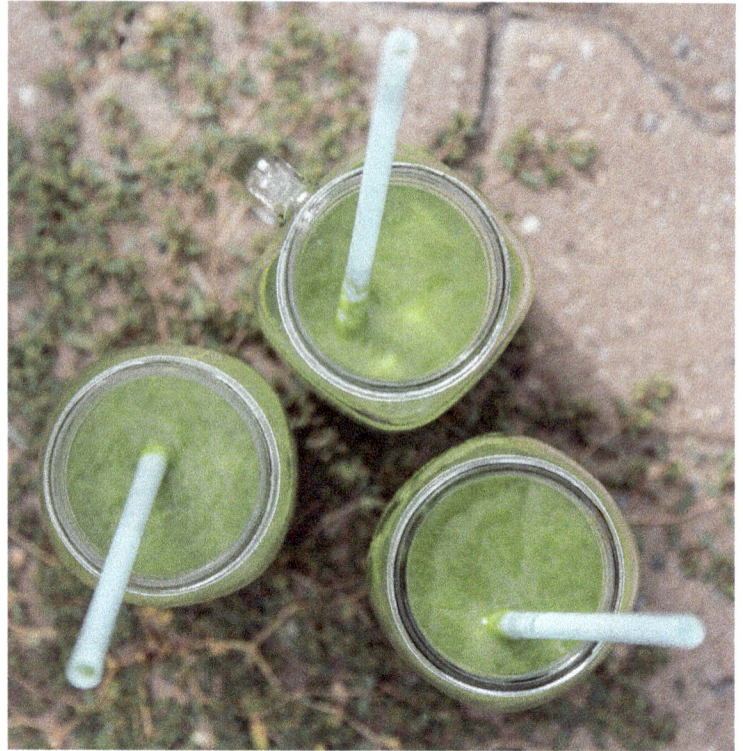

If you like, you can add the following supplements to the smoothie. Make sure to use the recommended daily dosage according to the bottle directions. Before beginning any supplement or vitamin, you should speak with your physician first.

- 1 daily dose multivitamin (Garden of Life is my favorite)
- Matcha green tea (as directed)

INSTRUCTIONS

Place all ingredients (including supplements) in a blender and blend until completely smooth. If it's just not sweet enough, add a few more pineapple chunks or one date.

* Use organic ingredients if possible.

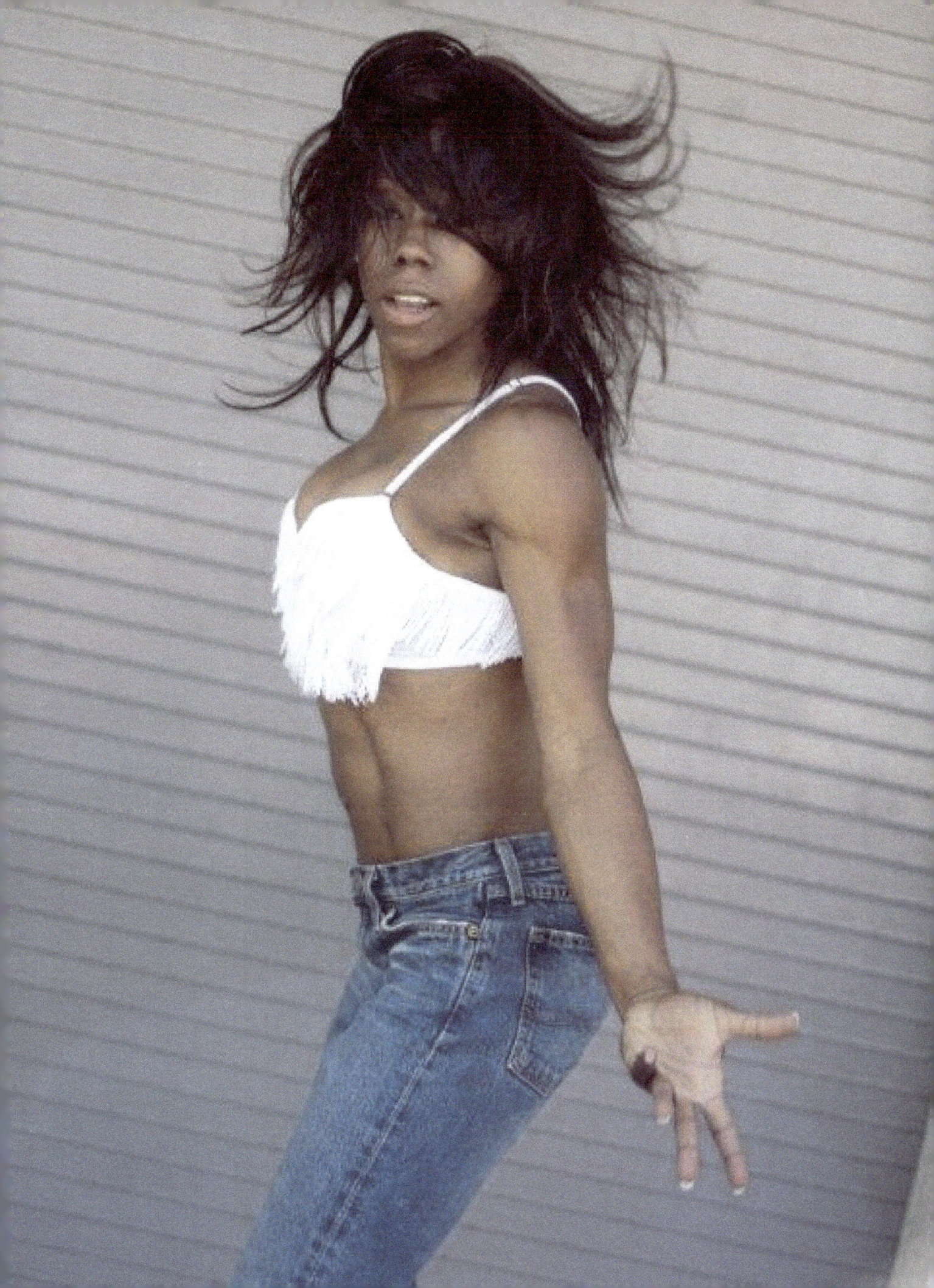

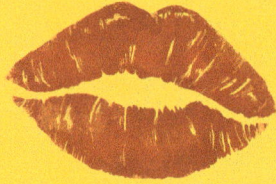

PART 3

MY BRAIN, HEART, AND BONE REGIMEN

HEART HEALTH

The sad reality is that heart disease is the leading cause of death for both men and women in America, killing approximately 610,000 people every year.

Many minority groups are at an even greater risk of developing heart disease; for example, nearly half of African American adults have some form of cardiovascular disease, such as heart attack or stroke. Most people disregard or even dismiss these looming statistics, believing it will not happen to them. As a result, they fail to take preventive measures to avoid this common but often unnecessary fate.

EXERCISE AND HEART HEALTH

Living a sedentary life puts you at a greater risk of dying from heart disease. The heart is a muscle, and just like your biceps or calves, it needs exercise to stay strong and healthy. You probably already know that unused muscles become weak and atrophy. Not only will neglecting physical activity result in a sluggish cardiovascular system, but a frail heart muscle will also be incapable of pumping enough nutrient-rich blood to meet the body's needs. Other organs will subsequently be at risk for failure as well.

HOW MUCH EXERCISE IS ENOUGH?

As mentioned in Chapter 2, the 10-20-30 interval training study done with trained runners at the University of Copenhagen in Denmark showed that interval training results in an improved cardiovascular profile. The 10-20-30 interval training may consist of any physical activity in segments of 5, 10, 15, 20, or 30 minutes scattered throughout the day. The benefit is that you don't have to do all of your exercises in one session.

Also, scientists at McMaster University in Hamilton, Ontario, reported that 1 minute of high-intensity interval training within a 10-minute exercise session is beneficial for your heart.[1] Keeping exercise short and simple with interval training allows you to be productive in less time while receiving cardiovascular benefits if you're consistently consistent. The exercise can be simply walking; according to the American Heart Association, walking just 30 minutes a day for six days a week will cut your chances of a heart attack in half.

The most sustainable exercise program is one that weaves short segments of activity into your day.

MAKE EXERCISE FUN

Planning your daily exercise around enjoyable activities makes it easier to stick to a routine. One idea is to make exercise a regular family event by taking a 30-minute walk outdoors after dinner. Walking together is a great way to connect with family while staying healthy at the same time! If you and your family want to maximize the exercise benefits, speed up the pace intermittently throughout the walk or incorporate calisthenics (jumping jacks, lunges, burpees, squats, high-knee marches). You can also include the 10-20-30 interval training. Be creative!

If you cannot exercise outside, you can walk, skip, or march around the house or couch for 30 minutes using the 10-20-30 routine. If you have stairs at home, you can complete my stair workout (as described in Chapter 5). Make sure you keep a steady pace. Any activity is acceptable as long as it increases your heart rate.

NUTRITION AND YOUR HEART

As we have established in previous chapters, nutrition has a significant impact on your heart health. To help you build a heart-healthy diet, I recommend that you consume foods from the following list each day:

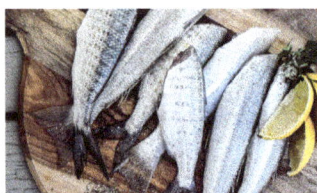

Fish

Wild-caught salmon, herring, trout, tuna

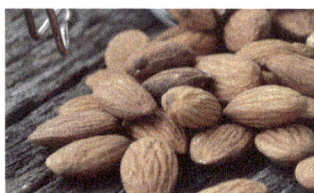

Nuts

Almonds, walnuts

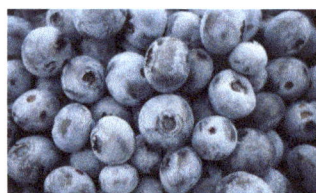

Berries

Blueberries, strawberries, raspberries, goji berries, acai berries

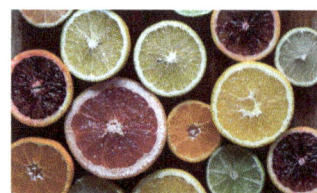

Fruits

Oranges, grapefruit, papaya, avocado

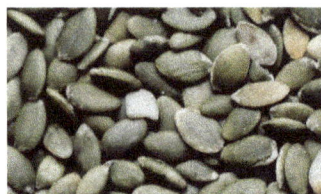

Seeds

Flaxseed, chia seeds, hemp seeds, pumpkin seeds

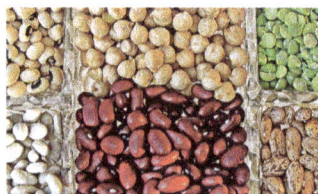

Legumes

Edamame beans, green beans, kidney beans, lentils, chickpeas, black-eyed peas

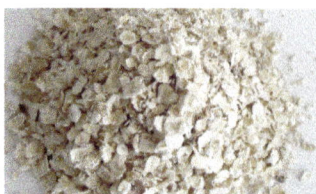

Grains

Oats, oat bran

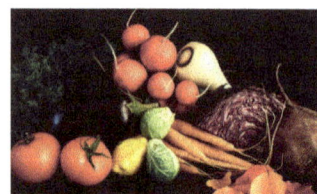

Vegetables

Red, yellow, orange, dark green leafy varieties, spinach, asparagus, beets, broccoli, carrots, tomatoes, squash

BRAIN HEALTH 17

Did you know that exercising affects not only your body but your brain as well?

TRAIN YOUR BRAIN

Your brain contains an essential protein called brain-derived neurotrophic factor (BDNF), whose primary job is to maintain the health of existing brain cells and to stimulate the growth of new cells. Low levels of BDNF play a role in the development of Alzheimer's disease, dementia, accelerated aging, depression, and cognitive impairment.[1][2] Hence, the goal is to sustain adequate levels of BDNF to ward off mental decline.

One proven way to increase BDNF is to increase your level of physical activity. Researchers believe that higher-intensity physical activity correlates with increased BDNF production.[3]

To reap the benefits, you must follow a consistent exercise program. Therefore, I recommend sticking to some form of exercise. Remember, it's all about being consistently consistent!

FOOD FOR THOUGHT

"You are what you eat" is certainly an accurate statement when it comes to your brain health. By eating what I call "brain-healthy foods" that contain plenty of vitamins, minerals, and antioxidants, you will nourish your brain and protect it from oxidative stress. Compared to other organs in your body, the brain is the most susceptible to oxidative stress because it requires a considerable supply of oxygen to execute demanding metabolic activities. These metabolic activities ultimately create a toxic by-product known as free radicals. Once the production of free radicals overcomes the body's ability to detoxify itself, oxidative stress occurs. Oxidative stress can cause damage throughout your body, especially to your neurons and brain tissue. If your body cannot detoxify itself or repair the damage, then it cannot defend itself from disease. To counteract the harmful effects of free radicals, you should consume foods that are high in antioxidants.

INCREASE YOUR ANTIOXIDANTS

Antioxidants are your best natural defense against oxidative stress, but your body does not produce enough of them to neutralize all the free radicals. As a result, your body needs a daily supply of antioxidants from outside sources. (See the list below)

SAY YES TO HEALTHY FATS

Did you know that your brain is composed of a startling 60% fat? It's the fattiest organ in the body. In the prenatal period, your brain begins accumulating fats to assemble cell membranes and other critical structures. Fats are essential for optimal brain development and nerve cell messaging. However, you can't just feed your brain any kind of fat! Your brain requires a steady stream of healthy fats, specifically eicosapentaenoic acid (EPA) and docosahexaenoic acid (DHA), to work properly.

To make shopping a little easier, I have put together a list of foods with healthy fats in the left column and potent antioxidants in the right column. These foods will help you sustain and even improve your brain health.

Whole grains

Beans

Pomegranate juice

Green tea

Blueberries

Dark green leafy vegetables

Dark chocolate

Wild-caught salmon, tuna, trout, herring

Nuts—almonds, walnuts, pecans, cashews (eaten in moderation because a 1-oz serving can provide up to 196 calories)

Seeds—pumpkin seeds, sunflower seeds without salt, flaxseeds (do not buy nuts and seeds with added sugar and salt)

Avocados

BONE HEALTH

18

A common myth is that physical activity can lead to joint pain and arthritis. On the contrary, exercise is actually a common prescription for arthritis patients.

Physical activity helps to maintain strong joints and assists in weight loss. Every pound you lose equates to four pounds less pressure on your knees and six pounds less pressure on your hips; it's a double win! Increasing your physical activity will also strengthen the supportive muscles around your joints and improve your bone density, particularly if you practice some form of resistance training. You do not need to lift heavy weights or have access to a commercial gym to reap the benefits of weight training. By using resistance bands, you can help build your muscles and support your joints.

To avoid unnecessary injury, always start small and gradually build your way up to heavier resistances. You can begin your exercise regimen by incorporating a simple outdoor stroll each day. Walking is a safe and effective way to decrease pain and disability—and best of all, it's free!

WARM UP

For those who suffer from osteoarthritis (as I do), it is crucial to warm up before each exercise session. Warming up stimulates synovial fluid movement within your joints. The synovial fluid serves as a cushion that protects them from impact.

Before warming up, I take a hot shower and do some light stretching while the water hits all my joints. The warm water loosens and relaxes my muscles, making them more pliable. After my shower, I begin with 5–10 minutes of dynamic stretching, an active movement that takes my body through ranges of motion. When I have completed these initial steps, I am ready to start low-impact physical activity.

TRY CHAIR AEROBICS

When I feel increased knee stiffness or achiness, I incorporate more swimming or chair aerobics into my exercise routine. I perform my favorite chair aerobics exercise routine to the "Casper Slide" song from Chapter 3. I follow the instructions of the song, just like "Simon Says." For example, when the song tells me to hop, I do a seated jumping jack or jump up to a standing position. Then, I immediately sit back down and resume following the instructions in the song. In the section where it asks me "How low can you go?" I do tricep dips on the chair, or I walk my hands down to the floor to do push-ups. Then, at the end of the song, I do flexibility exercises like side bends, shoulder circles, and hip flexor stretches while seated.

Another excellent chair aerobics routine, the "Best Chair Exercise Routine Ever!" by Alexis Perkins, can be found on YouTube. I recommend doing this routine five times for a total of around 15 minutes. Just google "chair aerobics," and you will find a plethora of routines to follow on your computer or phone!

BUILD MUSCLE

Building muscle is not about packing on the biceps like a bodybuilder. It is about gaining functional strength that will improve your quality of life and help your body function optimally. You may not realize it, but everyday living requires muscular strength such as getting in and out of bed, walking up and down stairs, combing your hair, brushing your teeth, putting away the dishes, and bringing the groceries from the car into your home.

Muscle strength naturally will begin to decline around age 40; therefore, it is imperative to incorporate strength training into your regimen so you can avoid injuries related to muscle weakness. Weak thigh muscles put you at risk for knee injury, while weak back and abdominal muscles put you at risk for lower back injury and possibly chronic back pain.

> **TIP:**
> IF YOU WANT TO CHALLENGE YOURSELF, DOWNLOAD THE EXTENDED VERSION OF THE "CASPER SLIDE" AND DO IT THREE TIMES FOR ABOUT 20 MINUTES.

To strengthen your body, try these simple bodyweight exercises:

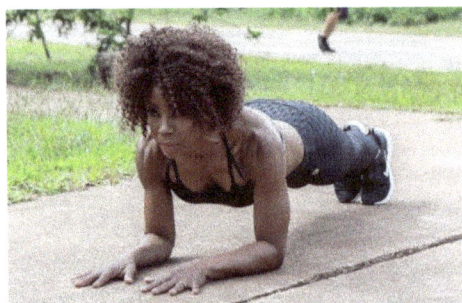

PLANK

I recommend "The Three-Minute Perfect Plank Workout" on YouTube because it targets and strengthens every muscle in the body at once. To get as much out of this exercise as possible, add variations like the side plank or one-legged plank.

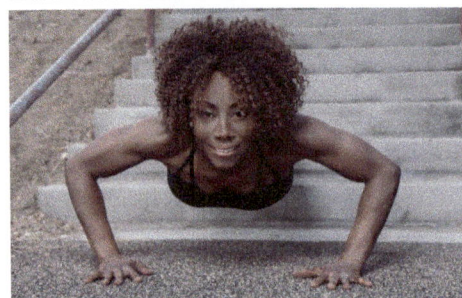

PUSH-UPS

Push-ups are one of the most basic and effective exercises that strengthen your chest muscles, shoulders, and triceps. Push-ups are also a terrific abdominal exercise because you need to maintain a tight core to perform them well.

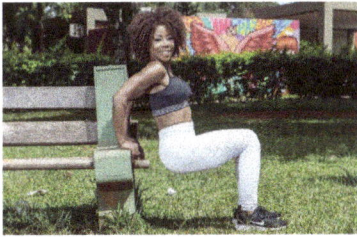

TRICEP DIPS

Tricep dips are a super simple way to strengthen your arms without having to use any equipment. All you need is a chair, bench, couch, or even a set of stairs, and you are good to go!

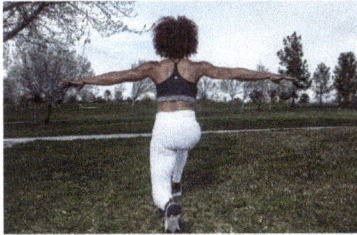

LUNGES

Lunges come in many variations that strengthen your lower body muscles, including walking, reverse, side, and front lunges.

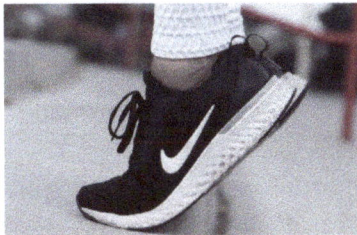

TOE RAISES

The next time you are standing in line or waiting for someone, take the opportunity to exercise your lower leg muscles by doing some discreet toe raises.

TIP:

A GREAT WAY TO INCREASE THE INTENSITY AND FURTHER STRENGTHEN YOUR MUSCLES IS TO INCORPORATE RESISTANCE BANDS. I RECOMMEND YOU BUY THE FIT SIMPLIFY RESISTANCE LOOP EXERCISE BANDS ON AMAZON. THEY COME WITH A FULL INSTRUCTION GUIDE!

DON'T FORGET TO STRETCH

Despite being one of the essential elements of physical agility and functionality, flexibility is the most overlooked piece of the fitness equation. What determines a person's level of flexibility is the health of their fascia, a connective tissue that encircles and supports muscles, organs, bones, ligaments, and tendons.

Many of us have poor postural habits, muscular tension secondary to stress, and limited mobility due to a history of injuries. All of these factors can cause or contribute to an increase of glue-like adhesions within the fascia. These adhesions restrict our body movements, causing our muscles to become inflexible and less productive.

To have healthy fascia, you must engage in regular movement and support your body's hydration needs by drinking enough water. A saturated, flexible fascia allows your muscles to stretch more, whereas a tight, dry fascia hinders your muscles from stretching, thereby increasing your risk for injury.

STRETCHING EXERCISES

Two of the tightest areas in the body are the hamstrings and hips. Try the exercises below to improve your mobility in these two areas:

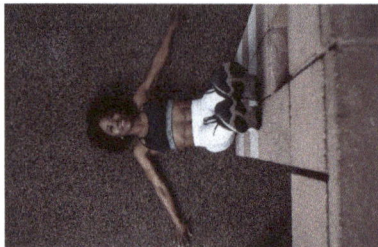

HAMSTRING WALL STRETCH

Lie on your back facing the wall with your butt touching the wall and your legs resting upward on the wall. Maintain the position for 30–45 seconds and then relax.

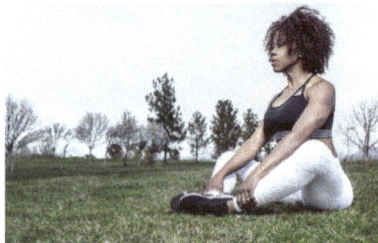

BUTTERFLY HIP STRETCH

Sit with your legs straight out in front of you. Then, bend your knees to pull your heels toward your pelvis. Drop your knees out to the sides and press the soles of your feet together. Maintain the position for 30–45 seconds and then relax.

MUSCULOSKELETAL-HEALTHY FOODS

As we age, we lose bone mass, thereby increasing the risk of osteoporosis. Osteoporosis is a process in which the bones become brittle and prone to fracture. For optimal musculoskeletal health, consume foods that contain a generous amount of calcium and vitamin D. Calcium and vitamin D work together to support and preserve your bones. Calcium's role is to build and strengthen bones, while vitamin D's job is to assist the body with calcium absorption. Good sources of calcium include milk, yogurt, kale, spinach, collard greens, broccoli, white beans, salmon, sardines, fortified calcium-rich nondairy milk, oatmeal, and orange juice. Vitamin D-rich foods include salmon, sardines, mushrooms exposed to sunlight, egg yolks, fortified dairy, and fortified nondairy milk and cereals.

> ## "WE WANT TO GO TOWARD MORE NATURAL, CLOSER TO THE EARTH, AND LESS-PROCESSED FOODS, WHILE AVOIDING FRIED AND PROCESSED FOODS, TRANS FATS AND CHARRED MEAT."
>
> **—NANCY CLARK, SPORTS NUTRITIONIST**

According to nutritionist Nancy Clark, processed foods, fried foods, charred meats, and trans fats increase inflammation. Many natural foods, on the other hand, decrease inflammation and are considered anti-inflammatory. A number of studies confirm that anti-inflammatory foods help reduce stiffness and joint pain.

A 1991 study that focused on 53 participants with rheumatoid arthritis concluded that a vegetarian diet without dairy and gluten may improve overall health and provide relief from symptoms like swollen joints, pain, and duration of morning stiffness.[1]

Another study in 2015 followed a group of 40 individuals with osteoarthritis who consumed a plant-based diet of fruits, vegetables, legumes, and whole grains for 6 weeks. The researchers found that the participants had improved physical function and a stark decrease in overall pain levels.[2]

Researchers have long believed that antioxidants can decrease inflammation in the body. One such antioxidant is green tea, which plays a role in reducing the severity of arthritis through its effects on the body's immune system.[3]

Furthermore, some studies have linked a high-fiber diet to a reduction of C-reactive protein (CRP), a known marker of inflammation associated with rheumatoid arthritis.[4]

Below is a list of the top anti-inflammatory foods. Color counts when it comes to combating inflammation, and the most vibrant fruits and vegetables are often the most powerful! When in doubt, choose darker, more vivid fruits and vegetables.

	Cherries		Flaxseed
	Blueberries		Kale, other dark leafy vegetables
	Blackberries		Collard greens
	Pomegranates		Broccoli
	Red peppers		Bok choy
	Wild-caught salmon, trout, sardines, tuna, herring		Extra virgin olive oil
	Oatmeal		Apples
	Turmeric root		Garlic
	Cinnamon		Avocado
	Ginger root		Green tea
	Walnuts		

DR. TRINA'S FAVORITE RECIPES

19

Here are a few of my favorite meals that incorporate various items from my pantry list in the Appendix. Try to use organic ingredients when possible, and feel free to add or subtract ingredients to your taste. These recipes serve as a foundation or guide to which you can add your very own flavor. For individuals taking medications for diabetes, heart disease, kidney disease, or other chronic conditions, consult your doctor before using LoSalt The Original. Each recipe serves 4–6 people.

DR. TRINA'S LASAGNA

INGREDIENTS

1 medium onion, chopped	Oregano
1 medium bell pepper, chopped	Chili powder
1 eggplant diced (can substitute zucchini or squash for the eggplant)	Garlic powder
	Onion powder
2 cups chopped portabella mushrooms	Simply Organic All-Purpose Seasoning
2 cups chopped shiitake mushrooms	Black pepper
Olive oil, for sautéing	LoSalt The Original
1 Beyond Meat Hot Italian Sausage ground up into crumbles	Organic, minced garlic
1 jar Sprout's Organic Pasta Sauce (No Salt Added) or Engine 2 Plant-Strong Organic Pasta Sauce or Dave's Gourmet	Tinkyáda Pasta Joy Brown Rice Lasagne noodles (9 noodles depending on how many layers you want)
Basil	So Delicious Cheddar Shreds and Mozzarella Shreds

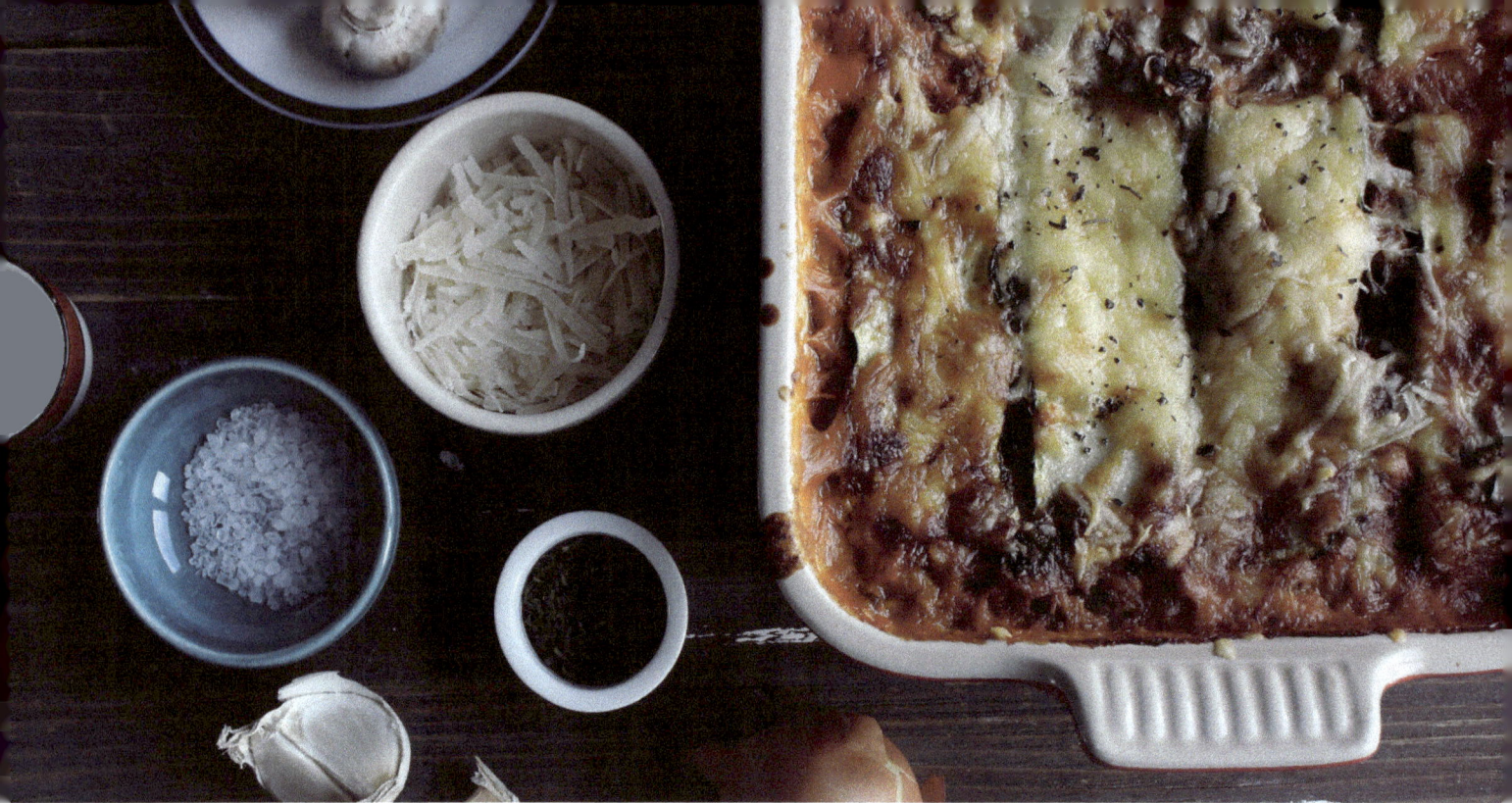

INSTRUCTIONS

- Sauté crumbled sausage with all vegetables. Add all seasonings. Cook until done.

- Add the jar of pasta sauce and stir. Simmer on low for 10 minutes, then taste to ensure it's fully cooked.

- Cook and rinse noodles as directed.

- Place 3 noodles on the bottom of a casserole dish. Save the remaining 6 noodles for the next two layers.

- Layer vegetable mixture over the layer of noodles. Sprinkle with a layer of each cheese to cover sparingly.

- Repeat noodles, vegetables, and cheese layers twice.

- Bake uncovered at 375 degrees for 30–40 minutes or until the top is golden brown.

- Serve immediately and enjoy with a side of fresh vegetables or a mixed green salad.

A spicy alternative to Beyond Beef Hot Italian sausage is Field Roast Mexican Chipotle Sausage. If you do not like spicy foods, use Beyond Meat Beef Crumbles.

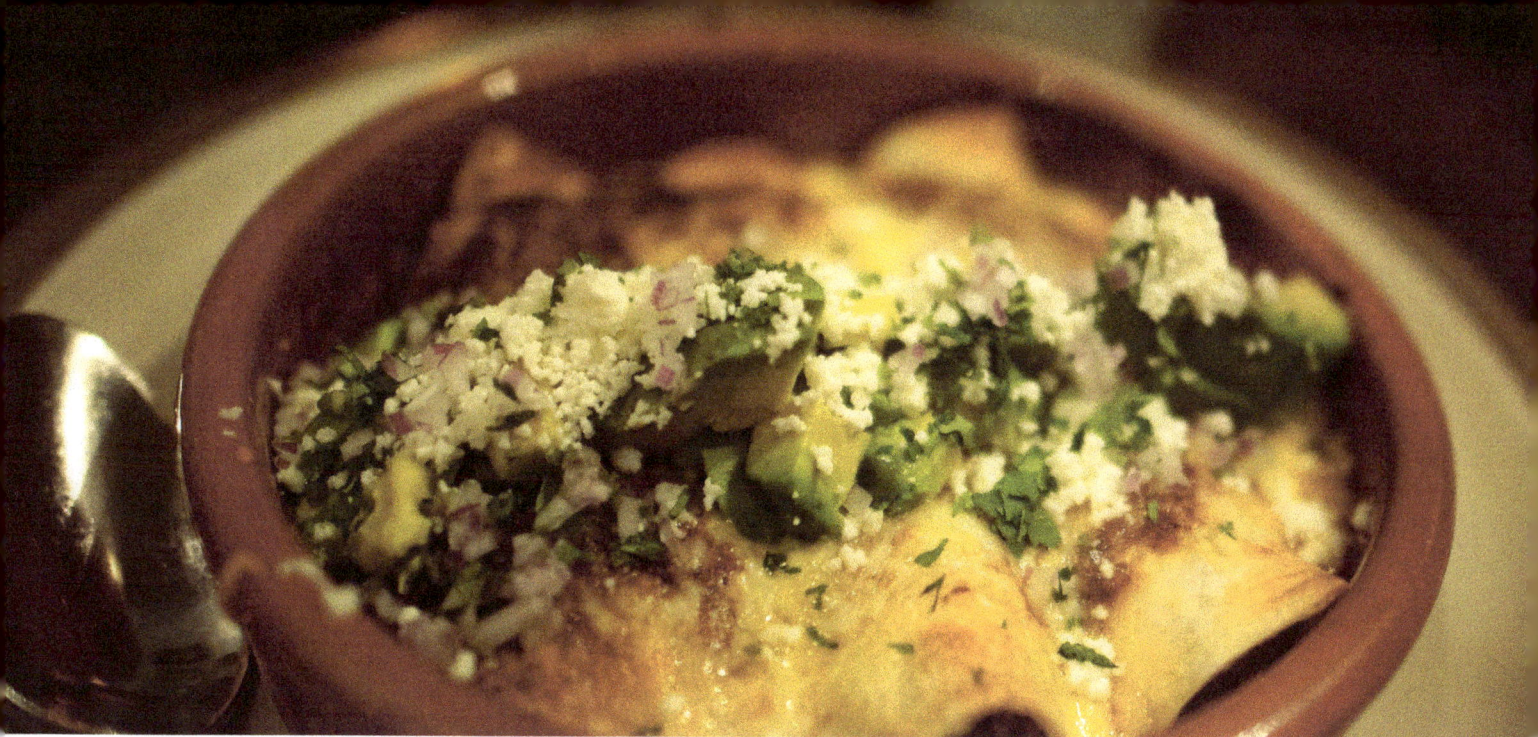

INGREDIENTS

1 medium onion, chopped

1 medium bell pepper, chopped

2 medium zucchini, diced

Olive oil (for sautéing)

Garlic powder

Onion powder

LoSalt The Original

Simply Organic All-Purpose Seasoning

1/2 to 3/4 bag frozen roasted corn

1–2 15 oz. cans black beans (no salt added), drained

Corn tortillas (I use approx. 6 Mi Rancho Organic Gluten-Free Corn Tortillas per can of beans)

1–2 jars 365 Organic Red Enchilada Sauce

So Delicious Cheddar Shreds and Mozzarella Shreds

Optional: The Jackfruit Company Smoked Pulled Jackfruit (jackfruit is a fruit with the consistency of pulled or shredded pork—it is sodium-free, cholesterol-free, and an excellent source of fiber)

DR. TRINA'S ENCHILADA CASSEROLE

INSTRUCTIONS

- In an oven-safe skillet, sauté the onion, bell pepper, and zucchini over low heat with all seasonings to your taste until tender.

- Stir in jackfruit, if desired, and heat through.

- In a separate skillet, heat the frozen roasted corn and black beans on low until hot. Add the beans and corn to the sautéed vegetables.

- Dice the corn tortillas into small square cubes and add to the mixture.

- Pour the enchilada sauce into the mixture until it's as creamy as you'd like, making sure to cover all the tortillas.

- Stir until the mixture is slightly soupy.

- Sprinkle one handful each of mozzarella and cheddar into the mix and on top to your liking.

- Bake uncovered at 350 degrees for 30–40 minutes.

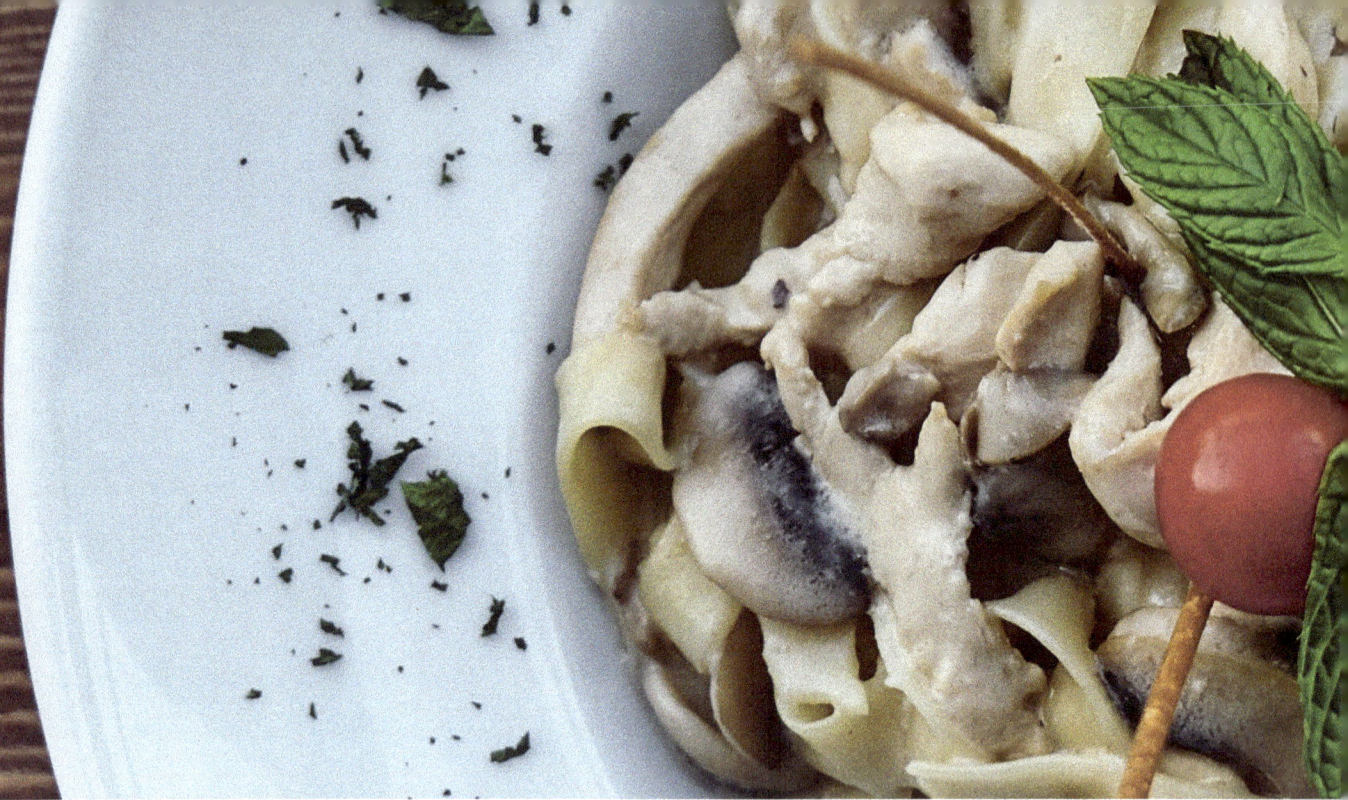

DR. TRINA'S BEEFLESS STROGANOFF

INGREDIENTS

1 medium onion, chopped

2 cups portabella mushrooms and 2 cups of shiitake mushrooms

Olive oil (for sautéing)

Simply Organic All-Purpose Seasoning

Black pepper

Onion powder

Garlic powder

1/2 bag frozen green peas

1/2 container Imagine Creamy Portobello Mushroom Soup

1/2 pack Gardein Home Style Beefless Tips (Optional)

1–2 tbsp. (approx.) Annie's Organic Vegan Worcestershire Sauce

1/2 cup (approx.) Tofutti Sour Cream

3/4 bag Tinkyáda Pasta Joy Brown Rice Fettuccine Pasta

INSTRUCTIONS

- Sauté the onion and mushrooms with all seasonings (to taste) on low heat until tender.

- Add peas, mushroom soup, and Beefless Tips along with Worcestershire sauce and sour cream. Cook on low heat for about 10 minutes or until the sour cream dissolves and the sauce turns light brown. The beefless tips and green peas should also be tender.

- In the meantime, cook the pasta as directed.

- Rinse and add the cooked pasta to the mixture.

- Stir the mixture until the sauce is well distributed.

- Serve immediately and enjoy with a side of fresh vegetables or a mixed green salad.

DR. TRINA'S MEATLESS MEATLOAF

INGREDIENTS

6–8 Amy's Organic California Veggie Burger Light in Sodium patties

1 yellow onion, chopped

1 green bell pepper, chopped

LoSalt The Original*

No-salt Italian seasoning

Onion powder

Garlic powder

Organic minced garlic

Simply Organic All-Purpose Seasoning

1/3–1/2 cup panko breadcrumbs

1–3 tbsp. tahini

1–2 tbsp. Annie's Organic Ketchup

2–4 tbsp. extra virgin olive oil (adds moisture)

Plain tomato paste (no sugar added)

Use sparingly.

INSTRUCTIONS

- Defrost the burgers until soft. Crumble them in a bowl with your hands.

- Lightly sauté the onion and bell pepper and add them to the burger crumbles.

- Season the burger crumbles with all seasonings.

- Add panko and tahini as a binder.

- Mix in ketchup and olive oil.

- Mold meatloaf into a mound and place on a lightly oiled baking pan.

- Cook covered with aluminum foil for 30–35 minutes, then uncover and spread tomato paste on top. Bake for an additional 10–15 minutes.

- Take out to cool and serve with a side of steamed vegetables and a baked potato. Enjoy!

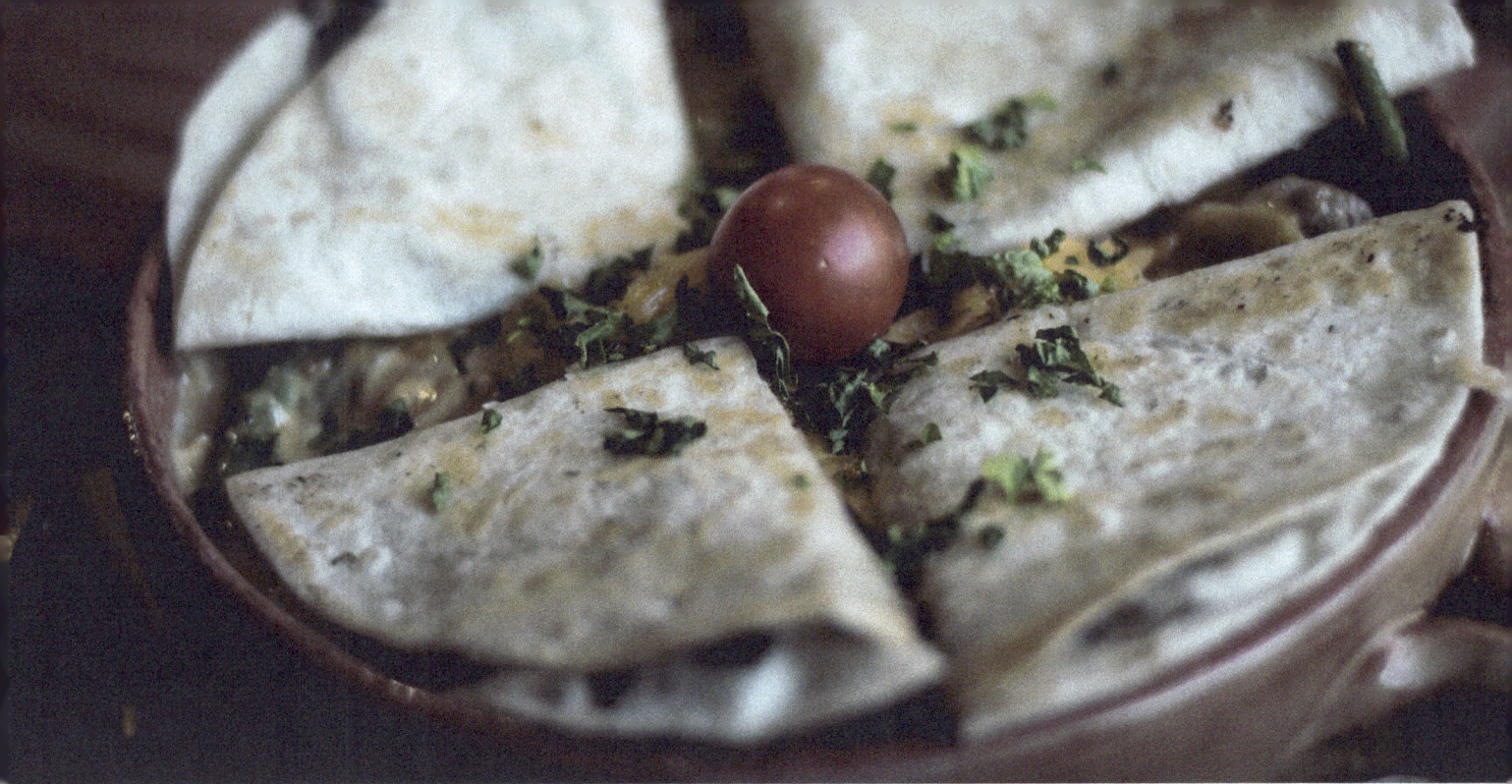

DR. TRINA'S BLACK BEAN AND YAM WRAP

INGREDIENTS

1–2 15 oz. cans salt-free black beans (drained and heated) or cook dry black beans from scratch

2 yams

So Delicious Mozzarella Shreds

Whole Grain California Lavash

1 tsp. Earth Balance Buttery Spread, for cooking

INSTRUCTIONS

- Peel the yams and cut into large cubes, then boil until soft. You can also bake the whole yams at 375 degrees until soft.

- Spread the yams on the lavash. Add the black beans and top with mozzarella cheese. Wrap the lavash to enclose the mixture.

- On medium heat, coat a skillet with the Earth Balance. Place the wrap in the skillet and let brown on each side.

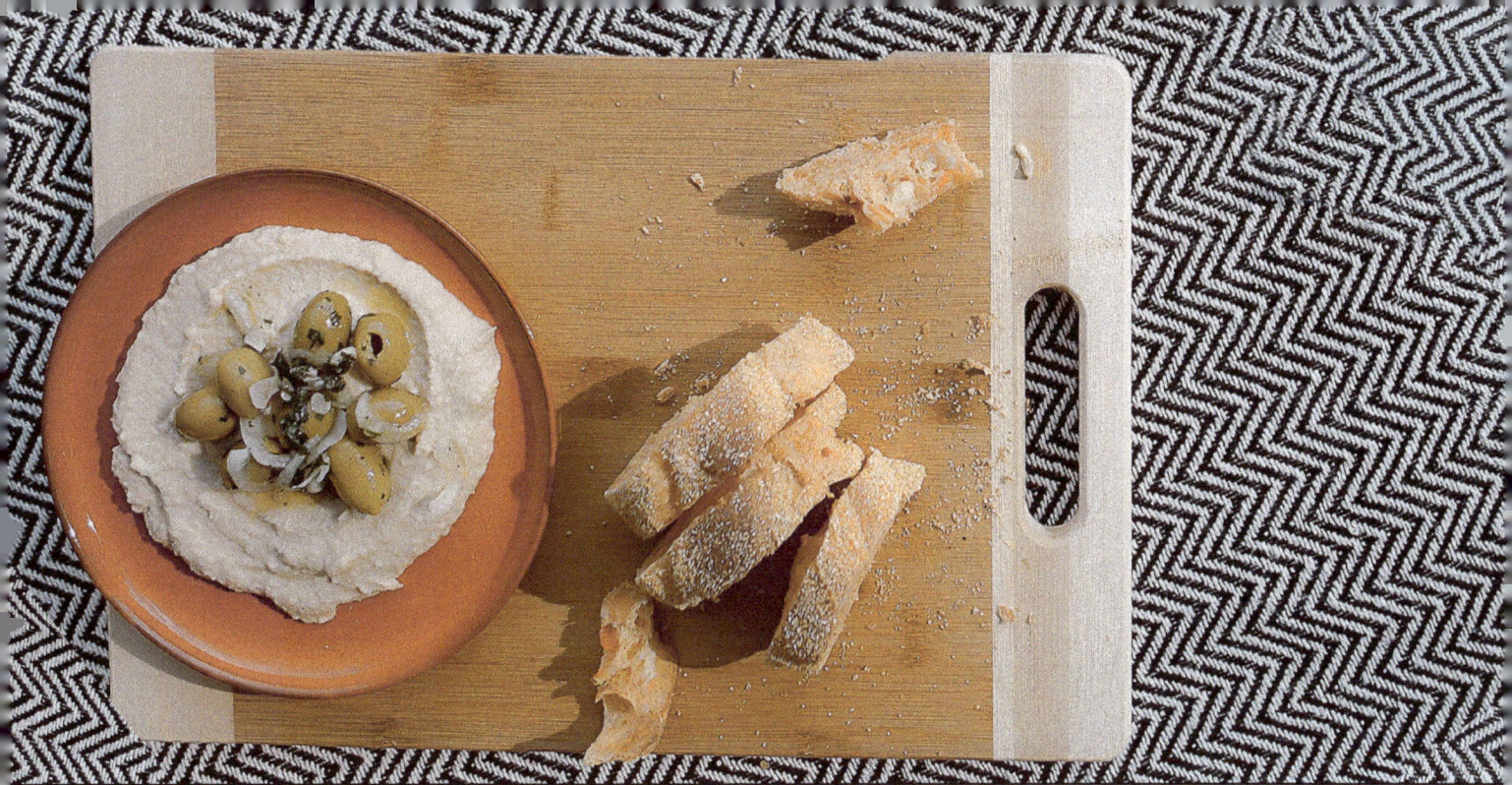

DR. TRINA'S GARBANZO BEAN MOCK TUNA: MY GO-TO QUICK LUNCH

INGREDIENTS

1–2 15.5 oz. cans 365 garbanzo beans (no salt added), drained

2–4 tbsp. Follow Your Heart Vegenaise

2–4 tsp. organic mustard

2–4 tbsp. organic sweet relish

1/2–3/4 medium red onion, finely chopped

INSTRUCTIONS

• Blend the garbanzo beans in a food processor or use a potato masher to mash them up.

• Add all other ingredients and mix thoroughly.

• Serve as a sandwich using Dave's Killer Bread Thin Sliced. Add a mixed green salad and some baked fries.

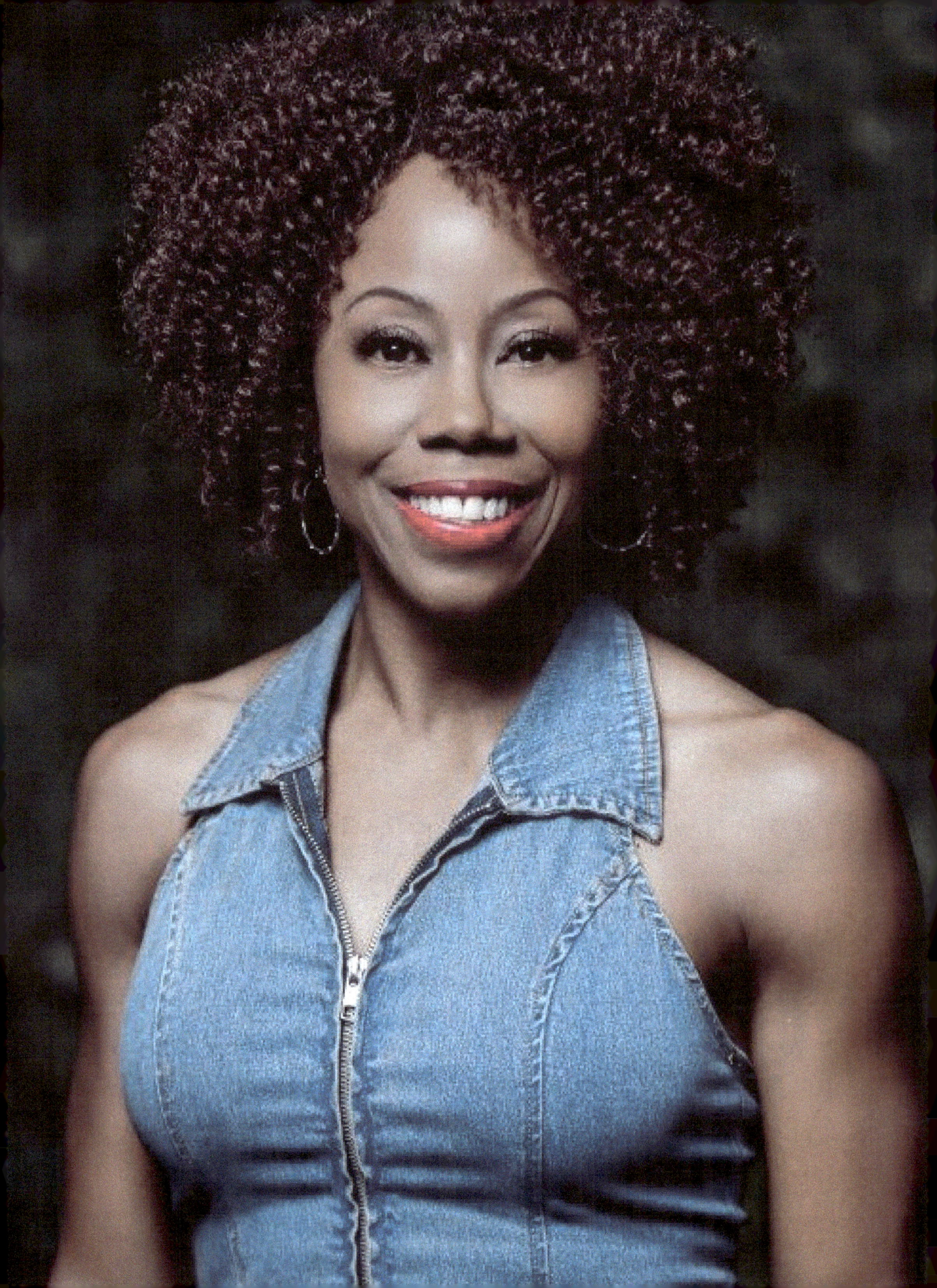

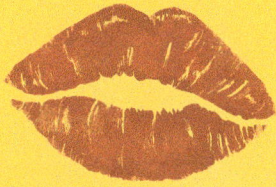

PART 4

DR. TRINA'S SECRETS

DR. TRINA'S TYPICAL DAY

20

Leading a healthy lifestyle comes down to finding routines that work for you. This chapter will show you what a typical day looks like for me and give you an idea of how my habits may benefit your health.

HABIT 1: DECOMPRESSING

After waking up in the morning, I invert on my Teeter inversion table. It is a terrific way to take the pressure off your joints and spine, thereby helping to alleviate stiffness and back pain. If you have a sedentary job that requires you to sit in front of a computer all day, you may find this especially helpful!

In addition to helping ease back pain, inverting on the Teeter inversion table is an excellent way to enhance the flexibility of your spine and relax your muscles.

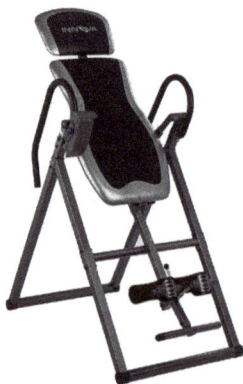

Other potential benefits include:

- realigning your spine and resolving the root cause of back pain

- decreasing pressure on your disks and facilitating rehydration between disks

- relieving painful nerve pressure through decompression

- reducing stress throughout the day and improving sleep during the night

It is important to note that the Teeter company recommends using the equipment only if you have a licensed physician's approval. There is an extensive list of medical contraindications for using an inversion table listed in the owner's manual. Please refer to the list of medical contraindications and confer with your physician before using this device. The most common contraindications are glaucoma, hypertension, heart disease, circulatory disorders, swollen joints, recent stroke or ischemic attack, and use of anticoagulants (including high-dose aspirin).

There are alternatives to the inversion table. Even though these alternatives are simpler, you should still consult your physician before engaging in any physical routine.

Fitness Ball Alternative: Lie across the ball with your back touching the surface. Then let your back stretch with your arms over your head. If you are able, try to touch the ground with your hands.

Yoga classes: Consider taking yoga because some of the poses require inversion.

HABIT 2: MEDITATING / PRAYER

When my body is relaxed and decompressed, I spend at least 5–10 minutes each day meditating. Performing this morning routine not only helps me clear my mind and get ready for the day ahead, but it also produces several other positive effects. Meditation can help:

- **Reduce Stress and Lower Cortisol**

A stressful life can lead to persistently elevated cortisol levels. Excessive cortisol levels are responsible for adverse side effects such as elevated blood sugar, suppressed immune system, digestive problems, heart disease, anxiety, depression, trouble sleeping, and foggy thinking. A 2011 study published in *The Journal of Alternative and Complementary Medicine* indicates that meditation can reduce stress levels and lower cortisol.[1]

- **Decrease Symptoms of Anxiety and Depression**

Studies have also linked lower stress levels to experiencing fewer symptoms of mental disorders such as anxiety and depression.[2][3][4] Moreover, studies have shown that meditation can help alleviate these conditions. Although the reason for this is not completely clear, it appears that meditation decreases the release of inflammatory chemicals called cytokines. As a result, mood improves as depression eases.[5] Another study compared electrical activity in the brains of people who practiced meditation with those who did not. For participants practicing meditation, the study revealed notable electrical activity in areas of the brain related to positive thinking.[6]

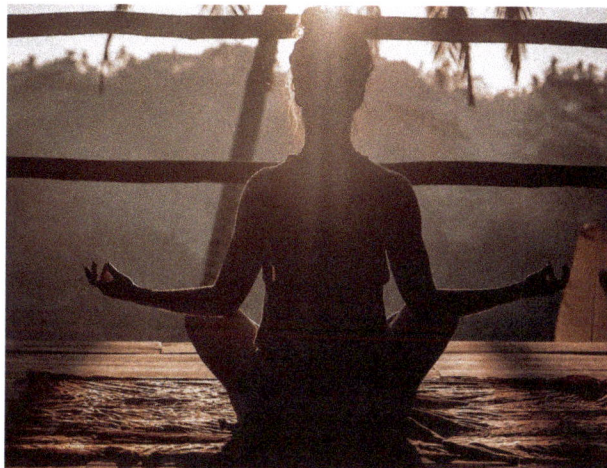

- **Increase Self-Esteem, Attention, and Focus**

Research suggests that consistent meditation has a positive effect on cognitive abilities such as self-esteem, attention span, and the ability to focus.[7][8]

- **Break Negative Patterns and Addiction**

Whether your self-defeating pattern involves binge eating, drinking, smoking, or even destructive relationships, meditation is a tool that can help you break this harmful pattern. Addictions are often complex and must be attacked from several angles. Increasing your self-awareness, focus, and positive thinking will allow you to understand your behavior better and regain control over your emotions and impulses. For most addictions, practicing meditation builds a strong defense against intense cravings.[9][10]

If you ask me, all these positive effects create a solid argument for spending a few minutes in silence every day!

Some possible benefits of meditation include pain control, improved sleep, decreased blood pressure, a more robust immune system, and even slowed aging. Prayer is just as beneficial as meditation; you can perform either one or both. Regardless of which discipline you choose, both meditation and prayer can lead to calmness and peace of mind.

If you are interested in learning more about meditation, you can find a wide variety of resources online and in app stores. One of my favorite apps is the Insight Timer.

It uses a gong sound that puts you in a calm, hypnotic state and helps you focus on your breathing. You can choose how fast or slow you want to breathe by adjusting the interval between inhaling and exhaling. I set the Gong Hanchi for 10–15 second intervals for a total time of 5 minutes. I inhale at the beginning of the gong sound, breathing in thoughts of positivity and fearless faith. I exhale at the beginning of the next gong sound, breathing out doubt, stress, fear, negativity, and toxicity. This intentional breathing helps to clear my mind and eradicate unwanted thoughts. It has also allowed me to increase the time I meditate because while in this hypnotic state, I lose track of time.

Other popular apps are Headspace and Calm. Both of these apps have valuable information and instruction on meditation, sleep, and relaxation.

HABIT 3: REHYDRATING

After meditating, I drink 20 oz. of room-temperature alkaline water with electrolytes. By drinking water at room temperature, I avoid brain freeze and actually consume more water daily.

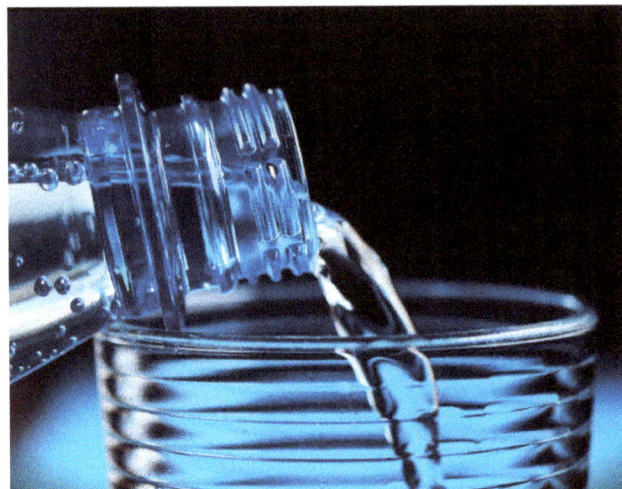

HABIT 4: DYNAMIC STRETCHING

Once I have rehydrated properly, I perform dynamic stretches for 5–10 minutes. Dynamic stretching is the use of flowing movements that take your body through ranges of motion—unlike static stretching (stretching in a stationary position).

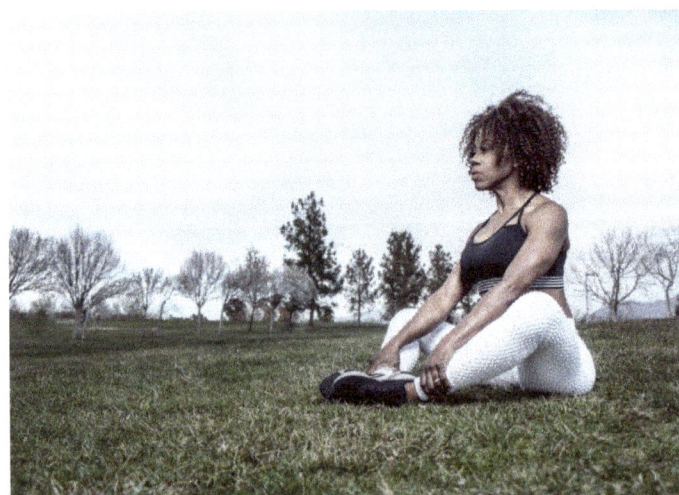

HABIT 5: STRENGTH TRAINING

After completing the dynamic stretches, I spend approximately 10–15 minutes working on my strength with resistance bands and bodyweight exercises like squats, lunges, push-ups, planks, and handstands.

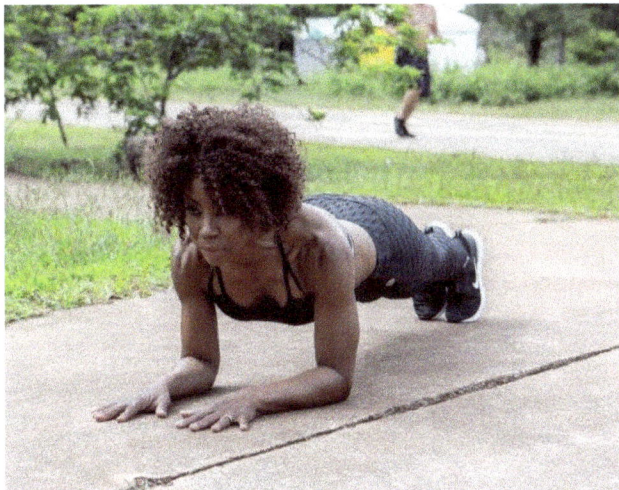

HABIT 6: DOING CARDIO

When my body is fully awake and energized, I am ready for my morning cardio. I typically spend anywhere from 30–40 total minutes broken up into 10–20 minute segments scattered throughout the day. In these segments, I perform various activities from part one of the book. To keep it interesting, I alternate between cardio exercises like biking, rowing, swimming, the "Casper Slide" dance, the "Cupid Shuffle" dance, the 7 Minute Workout app, and my stair workout.

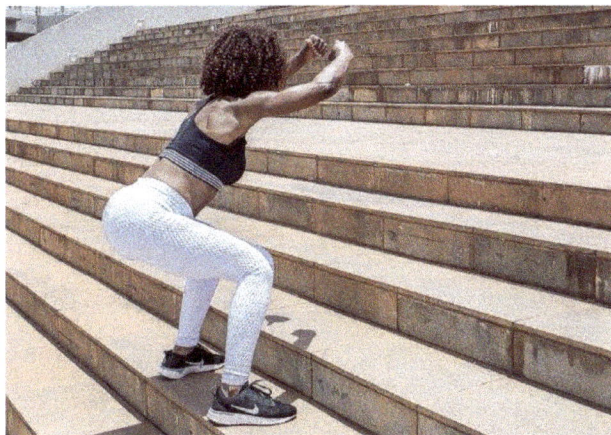

HABIT 7: SHOWERING

I try to find ways to make the most of each moment, so I always take the opportunity to stretch during my morning shower. A hot shower is a great way to relax and get your day started. It is also an ideal opportunity to stretch since the warm water loosens the muscles and increases flexibility.

HABIT 8: EATING BREAKFAST

Once I have exercised, stretched, and showered, I restore my energy levels with my daily superfood smoothie (see Chapter 15 for the recipe). In addition to the smoothie, I enjoy a bowl of oatmeal with a diced apple, banana, and cinnamon prepared in an Instapot. Preparation in an Instapot creates the perfect oatmeal every time that is creamy and sweetened with caramelized fruit and cinnamon.

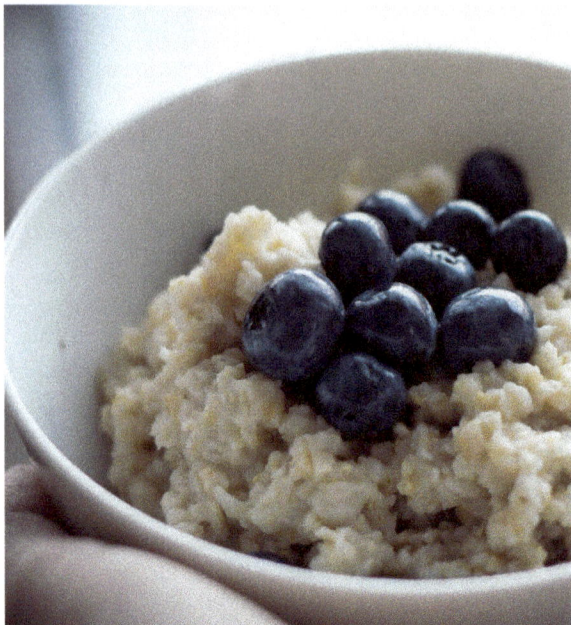

HABIT 9: INCORPORATING CONSTANT MOVEMENT

I try to stay active throughout the rest of the day by performing various stretches and exercises, such as toe raises, straight leg raises, and arm circles. I also incorporate activity by taking the stairs instead of the elevator (remember, going up one stair will burn 0.1 calories), parking farther away from stores, and pacing instead of sitting down while on the phone.

I always stay active one way or another, and I make it a point to exaggerate ordinary everyday movements to burn more calories.

HABIT 10: HEALTHY SNACKING

Unsalted nuts and seeds are the perfect snacks because they promote a healthy heart, suppress your appetite, and supply your body with a plethora of nutrients. So, when you are hungry and in a hurry, grab a handful of crunchable munchies like nuts or seeds. However, consuming too much can cause weight gain. One handful of nuts or seeds per day is all you need, which is about 1/4 of a cup. They are a great snack to have onboard to prevent you from driving through the fast-food line. In addition, they are one of the best foods to keep in your car for emergencies or when taking long road trips. Nuts and seeds won't spoil easily in the car. In fact, they can last up to six months to a year. However, it is important to store the nuts and seeds in a well-sealed, plastic, dry cooler to protect them from sunlight and temperature changes.

ALWAYS FIND A REASON TO KEEP MOVING!

TIP:
INCORPORATE N.E.A.T. ACTIVITIES WHILE WALKING THROUGHOUT THE DAY.

21

DR. TRINA'S TIPS FOR SUCCESS

Being determined to change your lifestyle is one undertaking, but actually succeeding is another feat that deserves special attention.

Life brings many unexpected events and obstacles that can hamper your efforts unless you have prepared effective strategies to overcome changes and challenges.

To make sure you come out on the other side as a champion, I have compiled a list of my very own tried-and-tested tips for success. As you consider which ones resonate with you, remember the guiding principles here: be consistent, and Keep It Short and Simple!

MENTAL STRATEGIES

THINK LIKE A WINNER

Think of yourself as an athlete. To improve your odds, you must enter this race with the mindset of a winner. I approach everything in my life this way—and let me tell you, it works!

SET YOUR GOALS AND MAKE A PLAN

Take time to define your goals and formulate a written plan to achieve them. Writing is a powerful tool to affirm your intentions, so make sure you put it all on paper. Make sure you intentionally create strategies and challenges to help you achieve your goals. For instance, when training for fitness competitions, I deliberately challenged myself to perfect my fitness tricks. I would make myself do a specific trick at least five times in a row without error. If I missed, I would have to start all over again. I kept a written record of my makes and misses. Doing the trick several times in a row without error gave me the confidence needed to achieve my goal.

To get on track with your fitness journey, I suggest setting up a time with a friend or two to dance together on FaceTime or Zoom for 15 minutes three times a week. No one would have to leave the comfort of their home. Download the extended versions of the "Casper Slide," the "Cupid Shuffle," the "Electric Slide," and the "Wobble" song for a total dancing time of at least 15 minutes three times a week. Consider getting a Fitbit to track how many calories you burn. After establishing consistency with your dance sessions, add calisthenics to make the dance more challenging. You and your friends can also create a dance routine. A long-term goal could be to meet in person once or twice a week to practice and refine your new dance moves.

This entire process can take place over 12 months, with the end of the year culminating in you and your friends entering an online dance contest. For example, I have participated in the Seniors Got Talent online contest. Check out the online talent videos with your dance crew to get excited about having fun while getting fit with a purpose. It's not about winning first place; it's about stepping outside of your comfort zone and challenging yourself to be your best.

Goal setting can also be utilized by parents whose children play sports. When my children were young, I would often see parents waiting near their children's practice at the track field, basketball court, soccer field, dance studio, or gymnastics facility.

While waiting, most of the parents talked on the phone or browsed social media. If you were to ask these parents about the importance of exercise, they would most likely agree that some form of activity is a good thing. Based on this premise, why not ask these parents to exercise with you while the children are training? It's a great way to make good use of your time. Don't let your phone and social media be temptations not to exercise.

Before practice is over, discuss dinner plans with those parents. Everyone knows it's very tempting to drive through a fast-food line after practice. Instead, suggest quick, healthy alternatives such as the black bean and yam

wraps and a salad or the garbanzo bean mock tuna with baked fries and a salad. Remind yourself, your children, and other parents that you all just did a fabulous workout, and now your body needs to be replenished with nutritious food. Use this time to inspire and motivate others to make wise choices concerning healthy living.

DECLUTTER YOUR MIND AND HOME

A messy home equals a messy mind, and the reverse is often true as well. Give yourself clarity and space to think by clearing out old junk that you do not need, both figuratively and literally. If cleaning out clutter feels like an overwhelming task, start slowly. Devote just 10 minutes a day to improving your physical surroundings and another few minutes to clearing your internal space using meditation.

Perhaps today's decluttering goals are to sort through that annoying stack of papers on your desk and remove at least one negative influence on social media that drags down your mood. Maybe tomorrow, delete junk emails, and finally donate those old T-shirts that you have collected over the years and have never worn. A little bit goes a long way, and you will soon be amazed at how much better it feels to be free of all those unnecessary things!

CHOOSE YOUR CIRCLE CAREFULLY

Surround yourself with people who believe in your goals and lead a healthy lifestyle. Limit the company of people who are not in alignment with your journey. Keep moving forward! Making these sorts of changes can be tough and lonely at first, especially if you find that most of your friends or family do not support your goals. Do not let this discourage you from putting your needs first. Stay strong, and rest assured your new lifestyle will attract a host of like-minded individuals.

FIND PEOPLE TO LOOK UP TO

Never be afraid of getting to know people who are more skilled than you in areas in which you'd like to excel. One of the biggest mistakes in life is to limit your opportunity to grow because you are afraid of being around people who are successful in areas you may find challenging. It's easy to feel bad about yourself and even become slightly jealous. Instead, try turning these negative thoughts into positive thoughts of admiration and inspiration that can propel you forward.

I encourage you to associate with people who know more than you about any given topic because it will only empower you and move you closer to your goals. You may have something valuable to teach them as well!

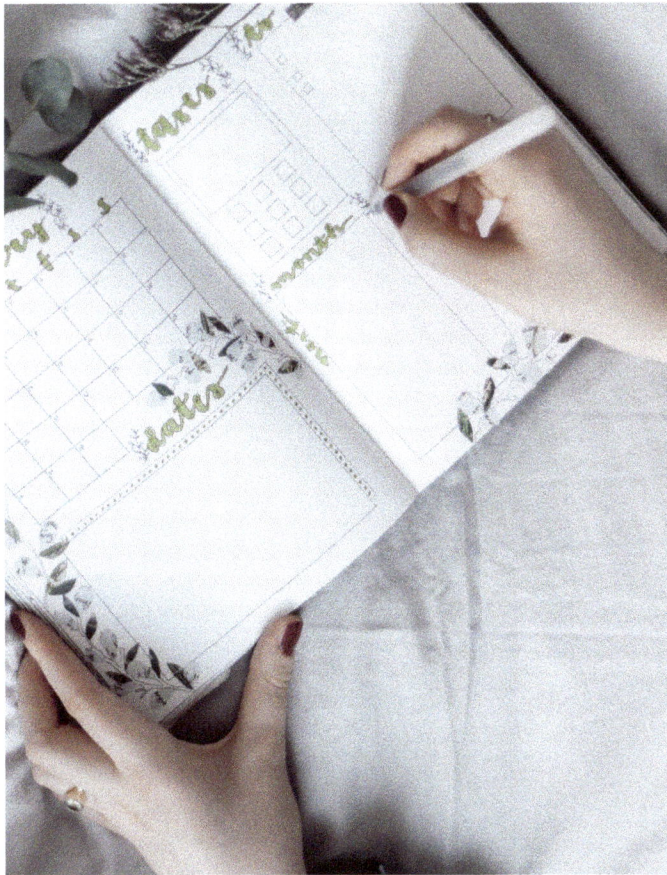

CREATE A TO-DO LIST FOR ORGANIZATION

Make it a habit to create a checklist of your daily goals, and make sure to keep the list with you at all times. Bringing it with you allows you to check off your daily accomplishments. More importantly, it will hold you accountable throughout the day. By establishing this habit, I am certain you will notice a big difference in how much you can accomplish with ease and efficiency in a single day.

MAKE YOUR WORKOUT AN APPOINTMENT

You wouldn't just skip an important doctor's appointment, would you? Start considering your workout to be a non-negotiable part of your schedule instead of something that falls to the end of your mental list of priorities.

REDUCE YOUR SCREEN TIME

Minimize the time you spend on social media and in front of the television. A good strategy is to set aside specific times to check your social media apps and limit how long you spend watching television or browsing the internet.

You will probably find that you have far more time than you think, and you will also see that there are better ways to spend your time than wasting it on mindless scrolling. You may even free up enough time to fit in a strengthening session with your resistance bands or a stretching session with the Stretch Out Strap.

LIMIT NEWS EXPOSURE

Staying up to date with current events is necessary, but no one benefits from 24-hour news exposure every day. Our brains can only process so much input at a time. With the omnipresence of social media and the internet these days, it's easy to get overwhelmed with information overload. Allow yourself a few minutes a day to get a quick update, and then resist the temptation to revisit any news sources for the rest of the day.

LAUGH AND SMILE MORE

Did you know that your physical and facial expressions have a substantial impact on your emotions? Similar to how walking with stooping shoulders and a downturned head can exacerbate depression symptoms, intentionally smiling and laughing can prompt your brain to produce endorphins that make you feel happy.

Positive energy begets positive energy. The more you consciously smile at people you meet or interact with, the more smiles you will get in return—and ultimately, the better you will feel.

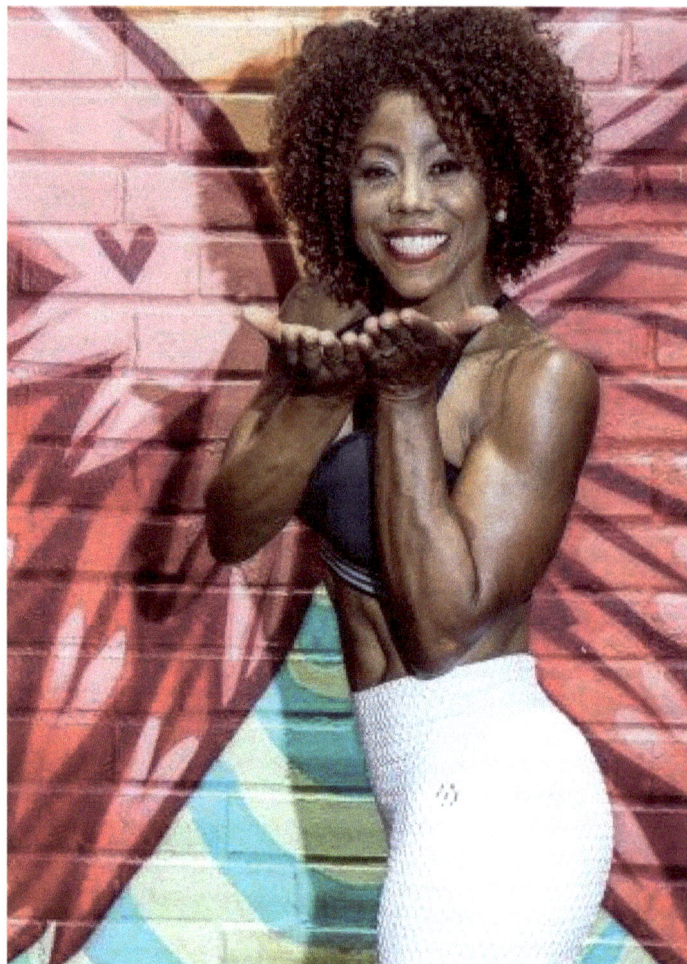

PRACTICE SAYING NO

While openness to new experiences and opportunities can be a positive trait, the ability to say no is equally important to your overall happiness and well-being. Listen to your gut and trust your mind and body when they indicate you have overextended yourself. Even though you may feel like you are letting someone down, take a step back and do what's best for you. You are not doing anyone any favors if you do not take care of yourself first, so make sure you balance your needs with those of others!

DO A GOOD DEED AND HELP SOMEONE

Helping someone in need can truly brighten your spirit. When dealing with a stressful situation, one possible coping strategy is volunteering your time to help others. In some cases, the best thing you can do to escape an emotional downward spiral is to get out of your own way. Deliberately removing yourself from a distressing situation will allow you to stop focusing on your problems and gain a new, healthy perspective.

JUST IF: INTEGRATE FITNESS

"JUST IF: Integrate Fitness" is a useful principle to keep in the back of your mind at all times. It means that rather than always being a scheduled event, fitness should be a consistent part of your life and incorporated into everything you do. Why not give yourself an extra reminder by hanging up a poster with the words "Just IF" or by wearing a heavy bracelet?

PIVOT YOUR MINDSET

Transform a negative situation into a positive one. We can't erase negative information we receive because the mind does not forget. However, we can reframe it and transform a liability into an asset. For example, when I sustained a knee injury in my 50s during the fitness competition season, I asked myself what I could do to maintain my strength and endurance. First, I cleared my mind, which allowed me to think creatively. Then I decided to purchase a rowing machine to use alongside my son's old skateboard. I rowed with one leg and let my injured leg ride along on the skateboard. This exercise routine allowed me to maintain both my strength and endurance. I also practiced handstands, which did not require the use of my legs. Subsequently, my handstands improved, and I was able to include more of them in my fitness routine.

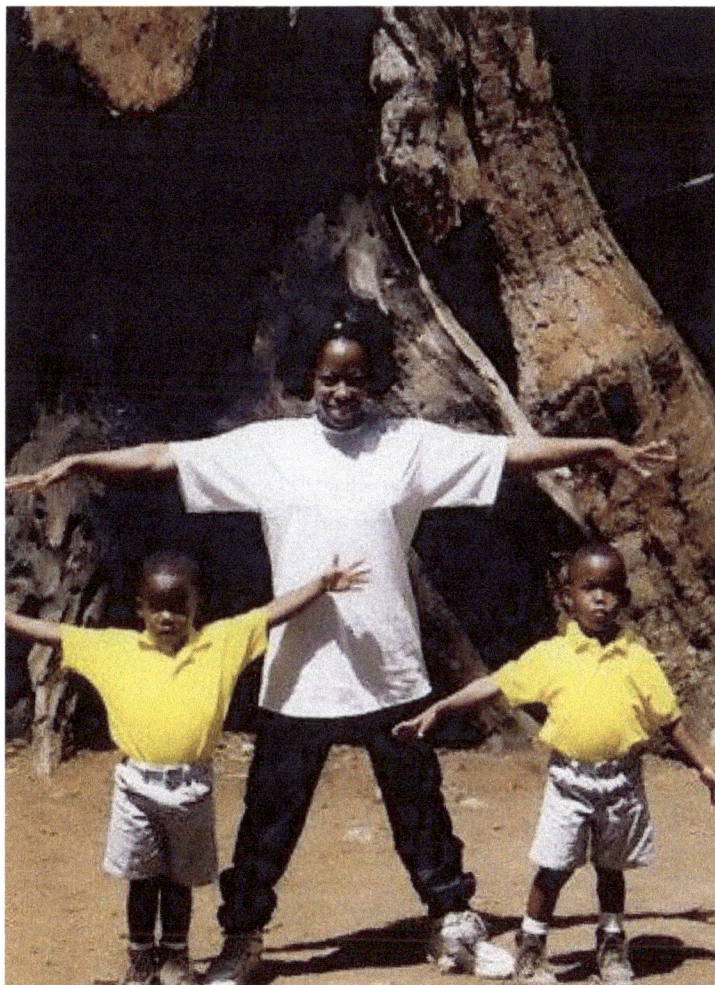

MIND-SOOTHING ACTIVITIES & EXERCISE

Your mind and body are two systems that are intricately connected and thus depend on one another's well-being to function optimally.

During stressful times, it's easy to fall into the trap of neglecting one of these crucial components of long-term fitness. Luckily, there are countless physically and mentally soothing activities that will help both your body and mind thrive.

HERE ARE SOME OF MY FAVORITE TIPS:

- Meditate outdoors in nature (try the Headspace app, Insight Timer app, or Calm app).

- Take up swimming.

- Start a regular yoga practice at a facility or online.

- Learn deep breathing (try the Breathe app or Insight Timer app).

- Get a relaxing massage.

- Take up a physically active hobby.

- Listen to soft music that makes you feel calm.

- Watch comedy to amp up your endorphins.

- Take an Epsom salt bath and surround the tub with vanilla or lavender candles.

- Go into the sauna, steam room, or shower to stretch and loosen your muscles.

- Put your legs up against the wall and relax.

PRACTICE DAILY STRESS-BUSTERS FOR WORK

Most people spend a large portion of their waking hours working, often confined to a desk in a hunched position that causes muscle pain and stiffness. Furthermore, men and women in all kinds of professions endure varying degrees of negative workplace stress that can have both physiological and psychological repercussions in the long haul.

Luckily, there are several simple ways to improve your work health and decrease your stress levels in the process.

TAKE MOVEMENT BREAKS

Make it a daily habit to take a few minutes after every hour of work to stretch and walk around. By doing so, you will return to work more focused and relaxed.

MINIMIZE CAFFEINE INTAKE

It's easy to keep going for the coffee machine when your energy runs low, but too much of a stimulant can cause unwanted side effects such as irritability, insomnia, anxiousness, shakiness, increased heart rate, and headaches. Reduce your coffee consumption and find more natural ways to raise your energy throughout the day. Consider taking brief breaks to do the following exercises: lunges, squats, toe raises, or tricep dips on a chair. You can also drink a smoothie in the morning and establish a regular supplement regimen that suits your specific needs.

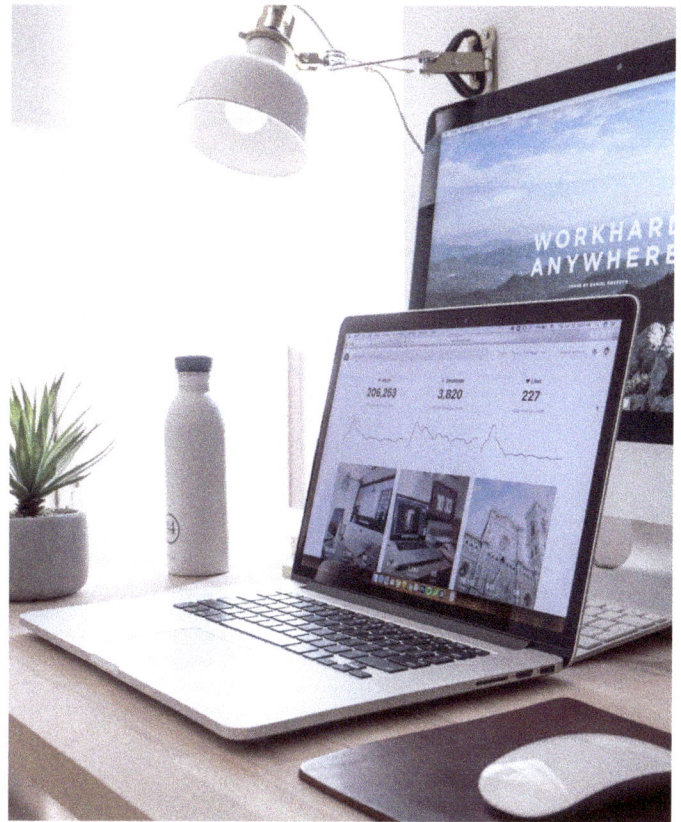

OPTIMIZE LIGHTING

Install full-spectrum natural daylight bulbs to create a better ambiance that can boost your mood. The natural light emitted from these daylight bulbs can also reduce eyestrain. If you don't have access to these bulbs, make sure your desk is near a window to allow in sunlight. Retract the window covering and adjust the blinds accordingly.

DECLUTTER YOUR DESK

No matter what your workspace looks like, make sure it is free of clutter and unnecessary distractions. Not only does a clean and organized workspace allow your mind to rest so you can focus on your task, but it also keeps materials accessible. As a result, you will avoid muscle strain caused by constant overreaching.

BUILD AN OASIS

If you cannot go to nature, let nature come to you! Create some form of an outdoor oasis in your workplace to reap the soothing benefits of nature. For example, place green plants on your desk or paint your home office walls blue to mimic the sky.

USE ESSENTIAL OILS

Research indicates that lavender can help alleviate conditions such as anxiety, insomnia, depression, and restlessness.[1][2] Put a small bottle of lavender oil in your desk drawer and rub a drop or two on your wrist and neck for a soothing effect.

CREATE POSITIVE WALL REMINDERS

Place positive affirmations and quotes on your walls along with family photos that bring you feelings of joy and love.

> ## "HEALTH IS NOT JUST BEING DISEASE-FREE. HEALTH IS WHEN EVERY CELL IN YOUR BODY IS BOUNCING WITH LIFE."
> —SADHGURU

UNMASK THE FACE OF FEAR

> ## "FAITH AND FEAR BOTH DEMAND YOU BELIEVE IN SOMETHING YOU CANNOT SEE. YOU CHOOSE."
> —BOB PROCTOR

"FEAR: False Evidence Appearing Real"

In nature, fear has a necessary and vital function to protect our body from external threats and keep us safe from harm.

Unfortunately, fear can also be misguided and unwarranted. In that case, it is a powerful and relentless enemy that keeps us trapped in dead-end comfort zones, locked into negative thought patterns, and enslaved to detrimental habits.

To combat fear, we must fight back by using positive affirmations, specifically out-loud self-talks. We can also seek the support of a friend who helps instill a fearless and confident mindset within us. One of my favorite affirmations is "Happiness, peace of mind, and fearless faith." I say it repetitively in my head or out loud until it becomes ingrained in my mind and soul.

> ## "FEAR KILLS MORE DREAMS THAN FAILURE EVER WILL."
> —SUZY KASSEM

INCREASE INTRINSIC MOTIVATION

There are two different forms of motivation: intrinsic and extrinsic. Intrinsic motivation is the kind that comes from within yourself, while extrinsic motivation comes from outside influences. In other words, you may be extrinsically motivated by the kind words of a good friend but intrinsically motivated by your positive self-talk.

It would be fantastic if you could always have both motivating factors in your life, but realistically, the only constant you can truly rely on is you. If you rely only on an external source, that source has the potential to break you down just as quickly as it can build you up. If you work on strengthening your intrinsic motivation, you will learn to rely on your sense of purpose and self-worth—a solid foundation that will always keep you standing no matter how hard the winds may blow against you. If others stand beside you and cheer you on, that's great. If they do not, you lose nothing. And ironically, you may even gain a greater sense of self-reliance!

You can raise your intrinsic motivation by envisioning your goals and keeping plenty of positive reminders and affirmations in your home, workplace, and car. Placing your favorite pictures of yourself throughout your home in areas that you pass by often can also encourage and inspire you. For example, I place my competition photos in my exercise room, kitchen, and bedroom. These pictures serve as constant motivation.

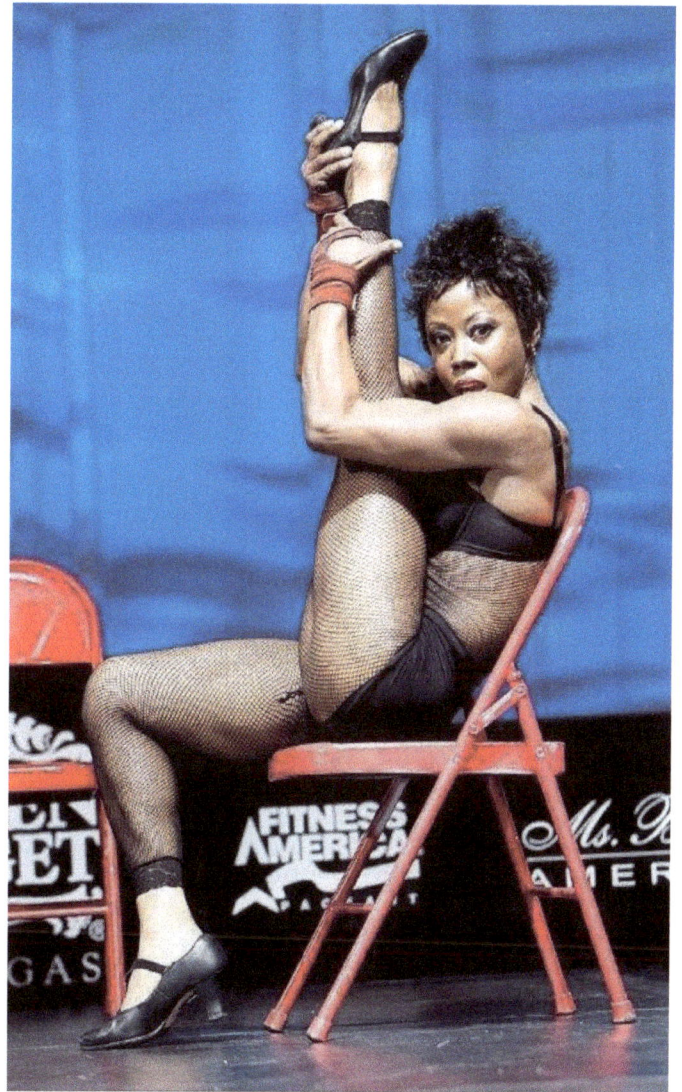

Whenever you feel motivation waning, return your inner gaze to your goals and keep your eyes glued to the prize!

CREATE A FIT HOUSE

The more opportunities you have to work out and the more reminders you have around you, the more likely you are to succeed on this journey!

The saying "out of sight, out of mind" certainly applies to fitness, so make sure you have workout items in sight every day as a reminder to exercise. Remember that even if you do just 5 minutes at a time, you have made progress. Small wins lead to big wins over time!

HERE ARE SOME TIPS TO HELP YOU CREATE A "FIT HOUSE" CONDUCIVE TO YOUR GOALS:

- **Create a fitness space** in the longest hallway (or any other suitable place) in your house. Include workout equipment like step boxes, an agility ladder for the floor, and a coat rack or hook on which to hang your resistance bands, Stretch Out Strap, and a jump rope.
- **Wear 1/2–1-pound wrist or ankle weights** while cleaning or doing other activities at home.
- **Create fitness stations** where you perform specific exercises like jumping jacks, squats, planks, and push-ups. Get creative and hang motivating reminders above the stations,

such as a framed poster saying, "Just do 5, and keep it moving!"

- **Hang a "sitting disease prevention" poster** with the words "Sitting Is the New Smoking!" as a reminder to keep moving. Instead of sitting on the couch while watching television, walk or skip around it.

By remembering the tips for success in this chapter and throughout this book, you'll be more likely to maintain a healthy lifestyle that supports your mental, physical, and nutritious needs. Choosing a simple method and a short time frame is a non-intimidating way to start practicing all of the K.I.S.S. tips you've learned until they become a habit. Each week, we'll focus on one theme and three tasks (a mental task, a physical task, and a nutritional task) to help you move forward with that week's wellness goals. By the end of this 12-week journey, you will have all of the necessary tools to achieve a healthy, sustainable lifestyle.

Ready? Let's get started now!

> **"WHAT YOU KEEP IN FRONT OF YOU, YOU'RE MOVING TOWARD."**
>
> —JOEL OSTEEN

> **"WE ARE WHAT WE REPEATEDLY DO. EXCELLENCE, THEN, IS NOT AN ACT BUT A HABIT."**
>
> —WILL DURANT

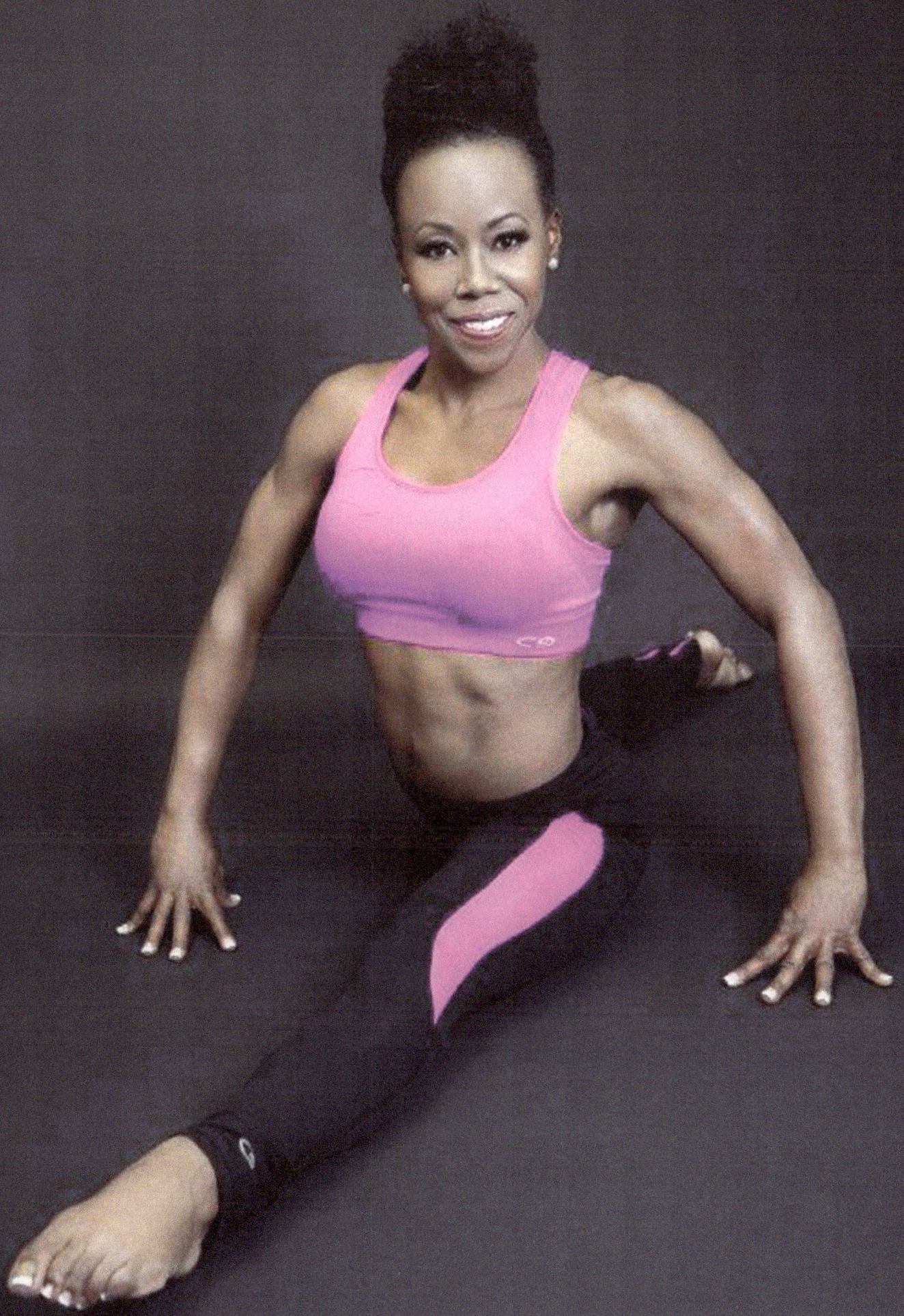

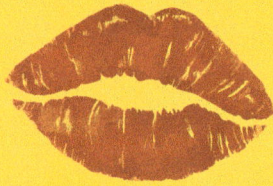

PART 5

MIND & BODY FITNESS

12-WEEK WORKBOOK

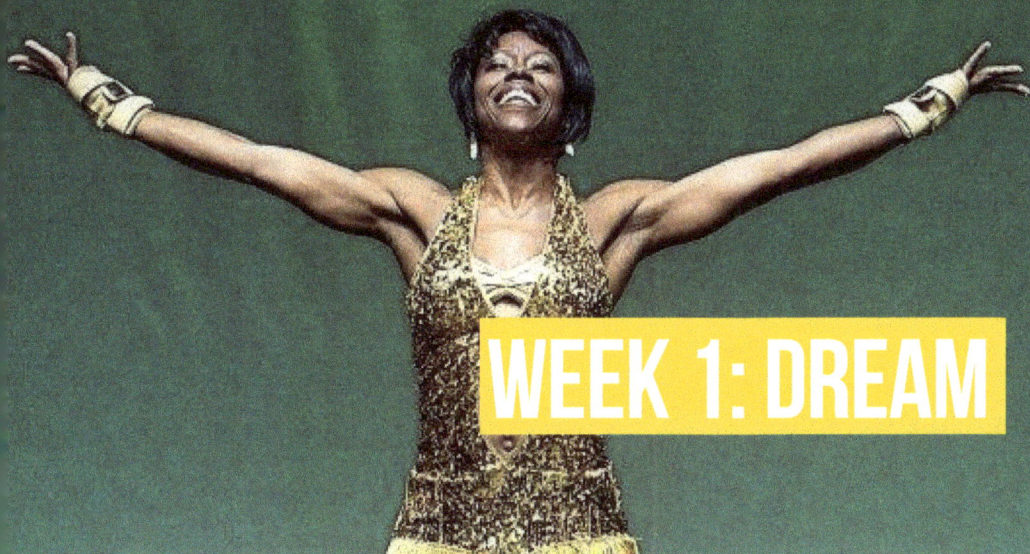

WEEK 1: DREAM

"DREAM SMALL DREAMS. IF YOU MAKE THEM TOO BIG, YOU GET OVERWHELMED AND YOU DON'T DO ANYTHING. IF YOU MAKE SMALL GOALS AND ACCOMPLISH THEM, IT GIVES YOU THE CONFIDENCE TO GO ON TO HIGHER GOALS."

—JOHN H. JOHNSON

WEEKLY MENTAL TASK:

Think back to your childhood or another time in the past, and find that thing that made you move your body irresistibly. Imagine yourself having fun without a worry in the world.

How does this younger version of yourself feel? Are you happy, confident, and full of energy? How is your relationship with your mind and body in this space? Is it different from now, perhaps in a positive way? How does this younger you view the world and the future?

Whether this vision was from your childhood or recent past is not significant. The essence of this exercise is to remember who you truly are, then feel the positive emotions that this past version of yourself was able to experience.

Once you can visualize this positive, healthy image, I want you to write it down. If you ever lack the motivation or inspiration to continue on your fitness journey, this will be your reminder of how you want to feel and why you started in the first place.

WEEKLY WORKOUT TASK:

Think about the previous exercise. Can you incorporate a past physical activity that used to ignite your body and soul? What small steps can you take right now to make this activity a part of your life again?

WEEKLY NUTRITION TASK:

What would your dream nutrition plan look like? Take a moment to think about which healthy foods you like and then plan your meals around those foods. For example, if you love sweet potatoes, google recipes that use sweet potatoes. There are a variety of ways to cook nutritious, delicious meals without sacrificing your health. If you focus on your favorite healthy foods, eating healthy will not be something you dread. Instead, it will be a different way of enjoying the good things in life.

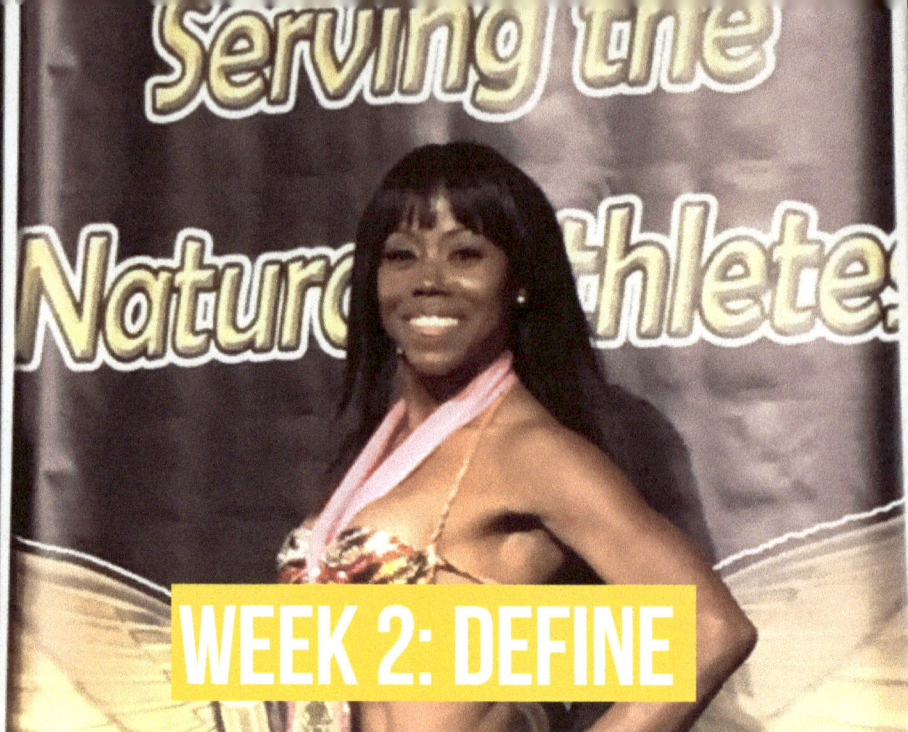

WEEK 2: DEFINE

> "FOR ME, FITNESS IS A PART OF MY EVERYDAY LIFE. BUT FITNESS DOES NOT MEAN HAVING BIG MUSCLES; IT MEANS BEING ACTIVE, QUICK, AND FLEXIBLE. IT CAN BE DEFINED IN MANY TERMS."
>
> —VARUN DHAWAN

WEEKLY MENTAL TASK:

Everyone has the potential to achieve a certain level of fitness, but the definition of fitness is different for everyone. This week, I want you to define your level of fitness. Maybe you want to begin the 10-20-30 program by walking 10–15 minutes in the morning and 10–15 minutes in the evening, or perhaps by jogging 10–15 minutes twice a day. If you seek an advanced routine, consider joining a running club whose members run together five days per week to prepare for an upcoming marathon. Whatever your fitness goal is, it is critical to define it thoroughly so that you have a clear image in your mind of what you are working to achieve.

This week, I want you to think about what fitness will look like for you. When you have a clear vision of your goals and your new routines, write them all down.

TIP:
REFER BACK TO PART 1 OF THE BOOK FOR IDEAS FOR YOUR NEW ROUTINES.

WEEKLY WORKOUT TASK:

Review your notes from this week's mental exercise.

Which healthy habits and physical activities have you envisioned to help you reach your goals? Pick one that you can implement in your life right now and make today the first day of your new routine.

WEEKLY NUTRITION TASK:

Define your portion size. What does your plate look like now compared to how it should look? Remember: use your hand to estimate your portion size. This week, aim to adjust your portion size and make sure that food from plant sources comprise the majority of your plate. When you put together meals, make your plate as colorful as a rainbow!

TIP:
IF YOU ARE INTERESTED IN PURCHASING MY PLATE, GO TO WWW.OPT2BFIT.COM OR TRINAWIGGINS.COM.

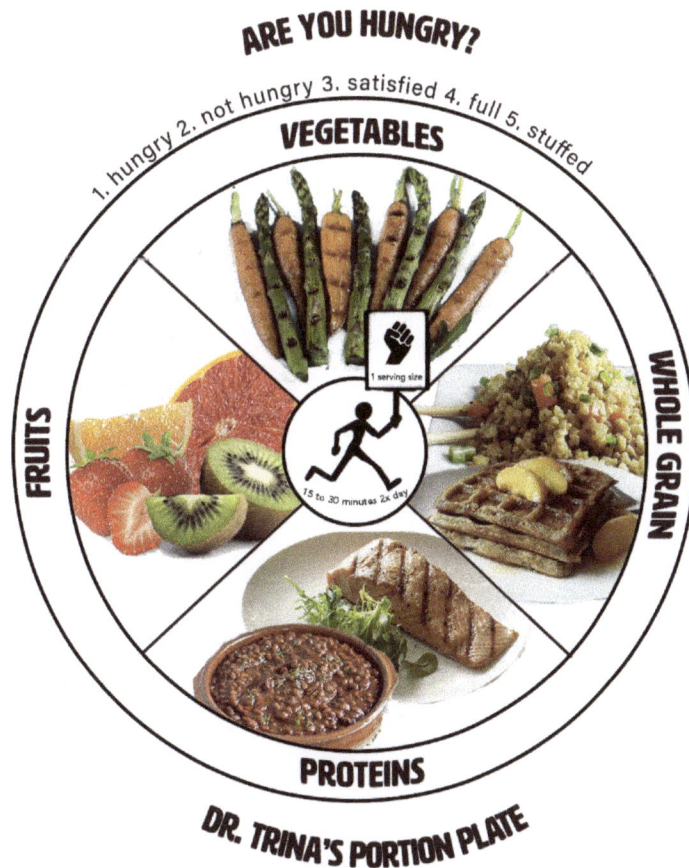

ARE YOU HUNGRY?
1. hungry 2. not hungry 3. satisfied 4. full 5. stuffed

VEGETABLES

FRUITS

WHOLE GRAIN

1 serving size

15 to 30 minutes 2x day

PROTEINS

DR. TRINA'S PORTION PLATE

WEEK 3: DIRECT

> "I CAN'T CHANGE THE DIRECTION OF THE WIND, BUT I CAN ADJUST MY SAILS TO ALWAYS REACH MY DESTINATION."
>
> —JIMMY DEAN

WEEKLY MENTAL TASK:

Think back to a time when you could have changed the direction and the outcome of a situation by viewing and approaching things differently. What was your state of mind at that time? What led you to think and act the way that you did? In what way(s) have you changed or not changed since then? How can you benefit from this experience in your future endeavors?

Think about it carefully and be honest with yourself. Write down your answers.

TIP:

IF YOU FEAR TAKING THE FIRST STEP WHEN IT COMES TO TRYING A NEW ACTIVITY OR RESUMING A PAST ONE, START SLOW AND GO OBSERVE YOUR NEWFOUND OR REKINDLED INTEREST IN ACTION. CONTACT THE LOCAL YMCA (1-800-872-9622, WWW.YMCA.NET/FIND-YOUR-Y), YOUR LOCAL CITY PARKS AND RECREATION, OR YOUR LOCAL AMATEUR ATHLETIC UNION (1-407-934-7200, HTTPS://APPLICATION.AAUSPORTS.ORG/CLUBLOCATOR/) TO FIND OUT WHERE YOU CAN JOIN YOUR SPORT. BEING AN OBSERVER CAN REMOVE SOME OF THE PRESSURE TO PERFORM AND INSPIRE YOU TO PARTAKE.

WEEKLY WORKOUT TASK:

This week, I want you to be candid with yourself as you put things in motion to begin your new sport. Identify specific tasks you need to accomplish in preparation to participate. You can google the necessary skillset for your particular sport. For example, if you are planning on joining a track and field club, you must increase strength and flexibility. To build strength, you can do squats, lunges, push-ups and planks. You can also wake up 30 minutes earlier to jog or run. Start with just 1 mile and gradually increase the distance. Upon returning home, stretch while taking a hot shower.

WEEKLY NUTRITION TASK:

Replace one cooked meal or dessert this week with a healthier alternative. If you haven't already done so, I highly recommend trying one of my favorite recipes from this book. I promise you will get hooked! You can also prepare your favorite meal with the ingredients listed in my Pantry Makeover (see the Appendix). To let me know how your meal turned out, feel free to hit me up on social media (@trina.r.wigginsmd on Instagram, trina.wiggins.79 on Facebook; @trinawiggins123 on Twitter) or through www.opt2bfit.com or www.trinawiggins.com!

TIP:

BE PROACTIVE AND CARRY SNACKS IN YOUR CAR SO THAT YOU ARE NOT TEMPTED TO DRIVE THROUGH A FAST-FOOD LINE. STOCK YOUR CAR WITH POPCORN, ALMONDS, GARLIC EDAMAME, WHOLE-GRAIN CRACKERS, OR GARBANZO MOCK TUNA (SEE RECIPE IN CHAPTER 19)

> "A SIMPLE LIFE IS NOT SEEING HOW LITTLE WE CAN GET BY WITH——THAT'S POVERTY——BUT HOW EFFICIENTLY WE CAN PUT FIRST THINGS FIRST . . . WHEN YOU'RE CLEAR ABOUT YOUR PURPOSE AND YOUR PRIORITIES, YOU CAN PAINLESSLY DISCARD WHATEVER DOES NOT SUPPORT THESE, WHETHER IT'S CLUTTER IN YOUR CABINETS OR COMMITMENTS ON YOUR CALENDAR."

—VICTORIA MORAN

WEEKLY MENTAL TASK:

Social media, an ever-present part of modern life, can be a blessing or a curse depending on how you use it. By limiting the amount of time that you spend on apps like Facebook and Instagram each day, you can avoid wasting time and energy. This week, I want you to minimize your social media usage by setting two specific times of the day to check your pages.

TIP:

TO AVOID GIVING IN TO THE SCROLLING TEMPTATION, SET ASIDE TWO TIME SLOTS FOR SOCIAL MEDIA, ONE FOR THE MORNING AND ONE FOR THE EVENING. CONSIDER TURNING OFF NOTIFICATIONS TO REMOVE THE TEMPTATION OF CHECKING THE APP WHENEVER YOU RECEIVE A NOTIFICATION.

WEEKLY WORKOUT TASK:

Your surroundings have the potential to impede or assist your goals. So this week, I want you to focus on creating a space that will be conducive to your efforts. Find a space in your home, such as the family room or garage, and start rearranging things. Clean out the clutter that you do not need and replace it with workout tools like resistance bands, a Stretch Out Strap, and a foam roller. You are much more likely to stick to your workouts if everything you need is right in front of you. Eliminating clutter and organizing your surroundings will direct you back to your fitness goals and free your mind from energy-sapping mental stress.

WEEKLY NUTRITION TASK:

This week, it is time to fight your cravings and declutter your kitchen. Flip forward to the Appendix to get started with my exclusive Pantry Makeover tips!

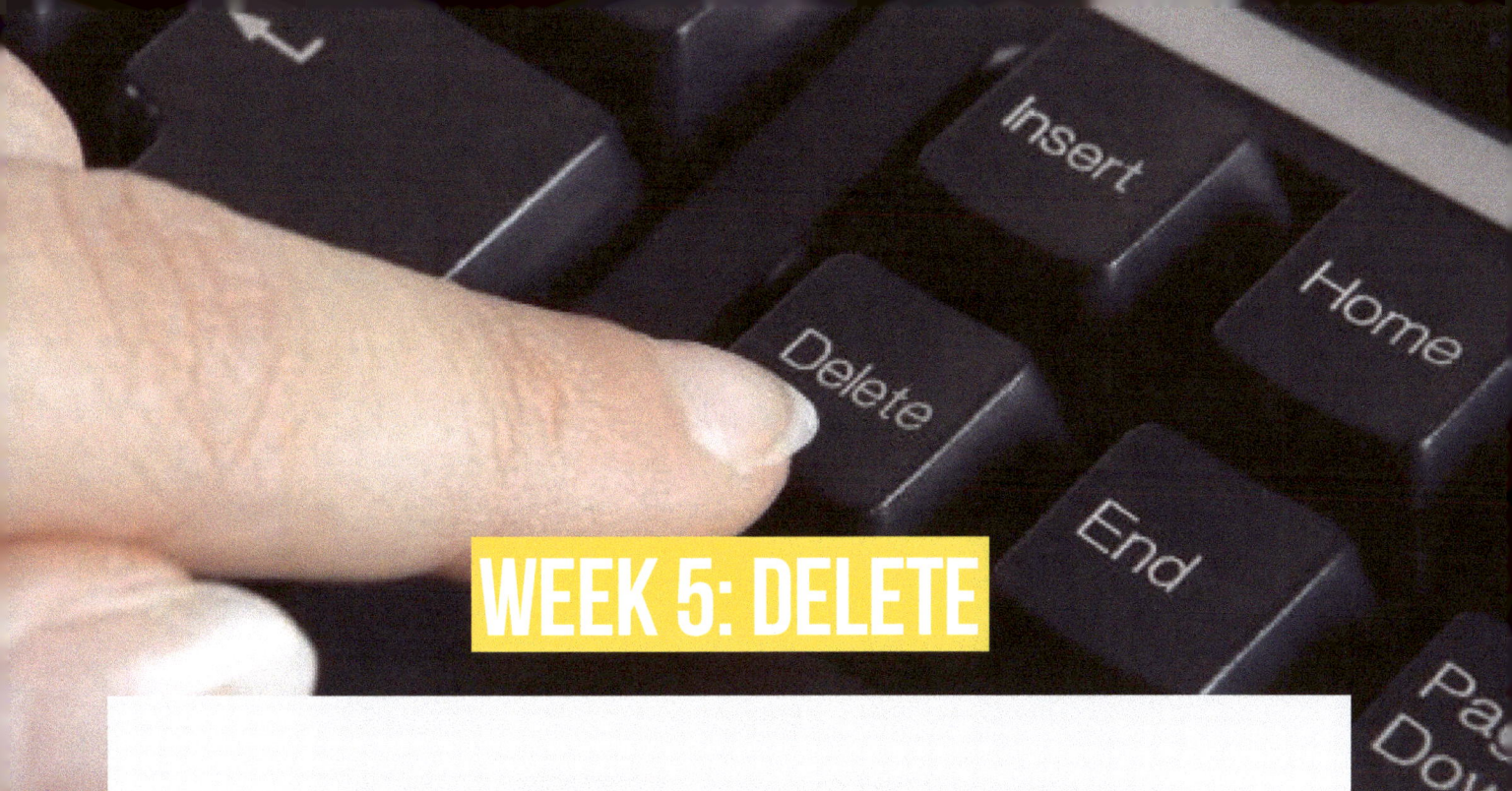

WEEK 5: DELETE

"DELETE THE NEGATIVE; ACCENTUATE THE POSITIVE!"

—DONNA KARAN

WEEKLY MENTAL TASK:

Surround yourself with people who align with your goals and support your journey. Avoid anyone negative and unsupportive. Delete all negative self-talk. Work on silencing that discouraging inner voice and replace it with positive verbal and nonverbal affirmations.

TIP:

TAKE A MOMENT TO DELETE ALL JUNK MAIL. TO PREVENT NEW JUNK MAIL FROM CLOGGING YOUR INBOX, INSTALL A SPAM BLOCKER, AND DON'T GIVE OUT YOUR EMAIL ADDRESS TO RETAILERS OR STRANGERS.

WEEKLY WORKOUT TASK:

This week is about continually moving from the time you get up until it's time for bed! Make a conscious effort each day to incorporate more N.E.A.T. (Non-Exercise Activity Thermogenesis) and do away with sedentary options like sitting or lying on the couch while watching the news. Instead, walk or skip around the living room while watching television and pace while speaking on the phone. Use your Fit Simplify resistance bands or Stretch Out Strap during your favorite show. Take the stairs instead of the elevator. Dance while cleaning the house. There are endless opportunities throughout the day to get your heart rate up and burn a few extra calories. So, get yourself moving and have fun while you are at it!

WEEKLY NUTRITION TASK:

Skip the soda! Soft drinks are a leading cause of excessive sugar intake. This week, I want you to eliminate all soda from your diet; instead, try this Dr. Trina-approved version!

Instructions:

Simply mix 1/4 cup of your favorite 100% juice and 3/4 cup of sparkling water in a glass, and voila, you have a super tasty and perfectly healthy soda alternative. Enjoy!

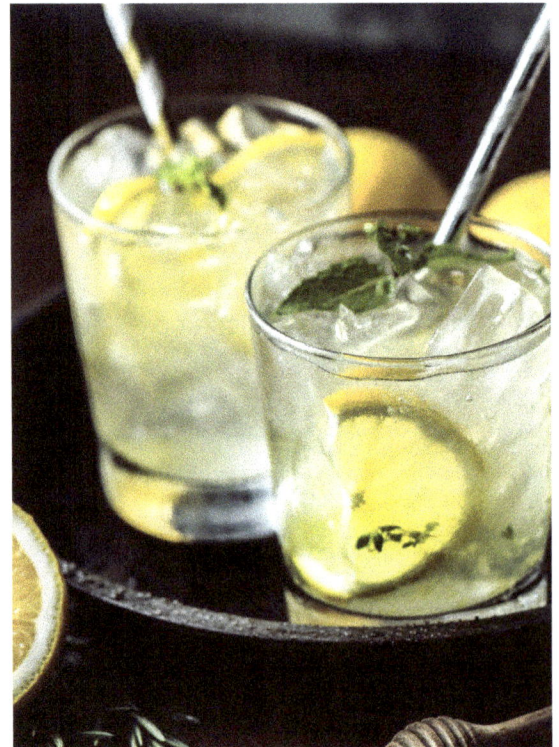

WEEK 6: DISCONNECT

"NOWADAYS WE HAVE SO MANY THINGS THAT TAKE OUR ATTENTION—PHONES, INTERNET—AND PERHAPS WE NEED TO DISCONNECT FROM THOSE AND FOCUS ON THE IMMEDIATE WORLD AROUND US AND THE PEOPLE THAT ARE ACTUALLY PRESENT."

—NICHOLAS HOULT

WEEKLY MENTAL TASK:

This week is about disconnecting and letting your mind rest. Limit the amount of time you spend in front of all screens, including your smartphone, tablet, laptop, and television. Reducing your screen time to a maximum of two hours a day (excluding work-related tasks) will increase the time you have to pursue your dreams and goals.

WEEKLY WORKOUT TASK:

Change how you transport yourself from one place to another. Walk or bike instead of driving and ditch the elevator in favor of the stairs.

TIP:
USE THE 10-20-30 METHOD WHEN WALKING TO BURN MORE CALORIES!

WEEKLY NUTRITION TASK:

Limit the number of times you eat out and instead cook meals at home. Doing so will lead to a vast improvement in your nutrition; your wallet will thank you as well.

WEEK 7: DECOMPRESS

"THE SECRET OF RELAXATION IS IN THESE THREE WORDS: 'LET IT GO!'"

—DADA J. P. VASWANI

WEEKLY MENTAL TASK:

Long-term stress is hard on the body. One of the best things you can do for your health is to learn how to decompress both physically and mentally. Instead of resorting to a glass of wine after work, treat yourself to a hot Epsom salt bath. Epsom salt can help improve sleep, relieve stress, relax sore muscles, loosen stiff joints, and relieve bruising, swelling, and sprains.

WEEKLY WORKOUT TASK:

Take a few minutes each day to decompress your spine (see Chapter 20). Try lying on your back with your knees bent and your feet flat on the ground. Then pull one knee to your chest for about ten seconds and repeat with the other knee. Lastly, try the Cat Stretch by getting onto your hands and knees and arching up your back. Google "Cat Stretch" for further information.

TIP:
TO GIVE YOURSELF A FULL SPA EXPERIENCE, USE A REJUVENATING FACE MASK WHILE BURNING SOME SOOTHING LAVENDER CANDLES AROUND THE TUB!

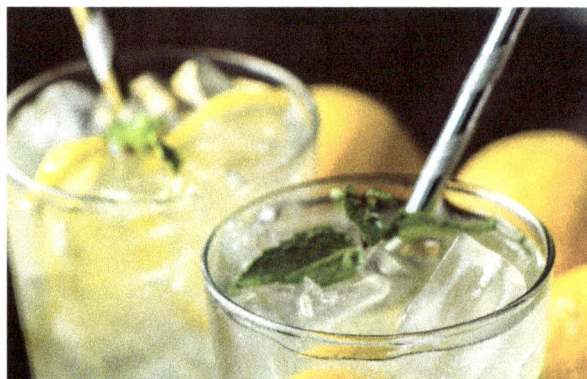

WEEKLY NUTRITION TASK:

Give your body a natural health boost by mixing a detox drink with three simple ingredients: water, lemons, and ginger (or just lemon and water). Commit to drinking half of your body weight in ounces of water each day to make sure your body stays fully hydrated.

WEEK 8: DEED

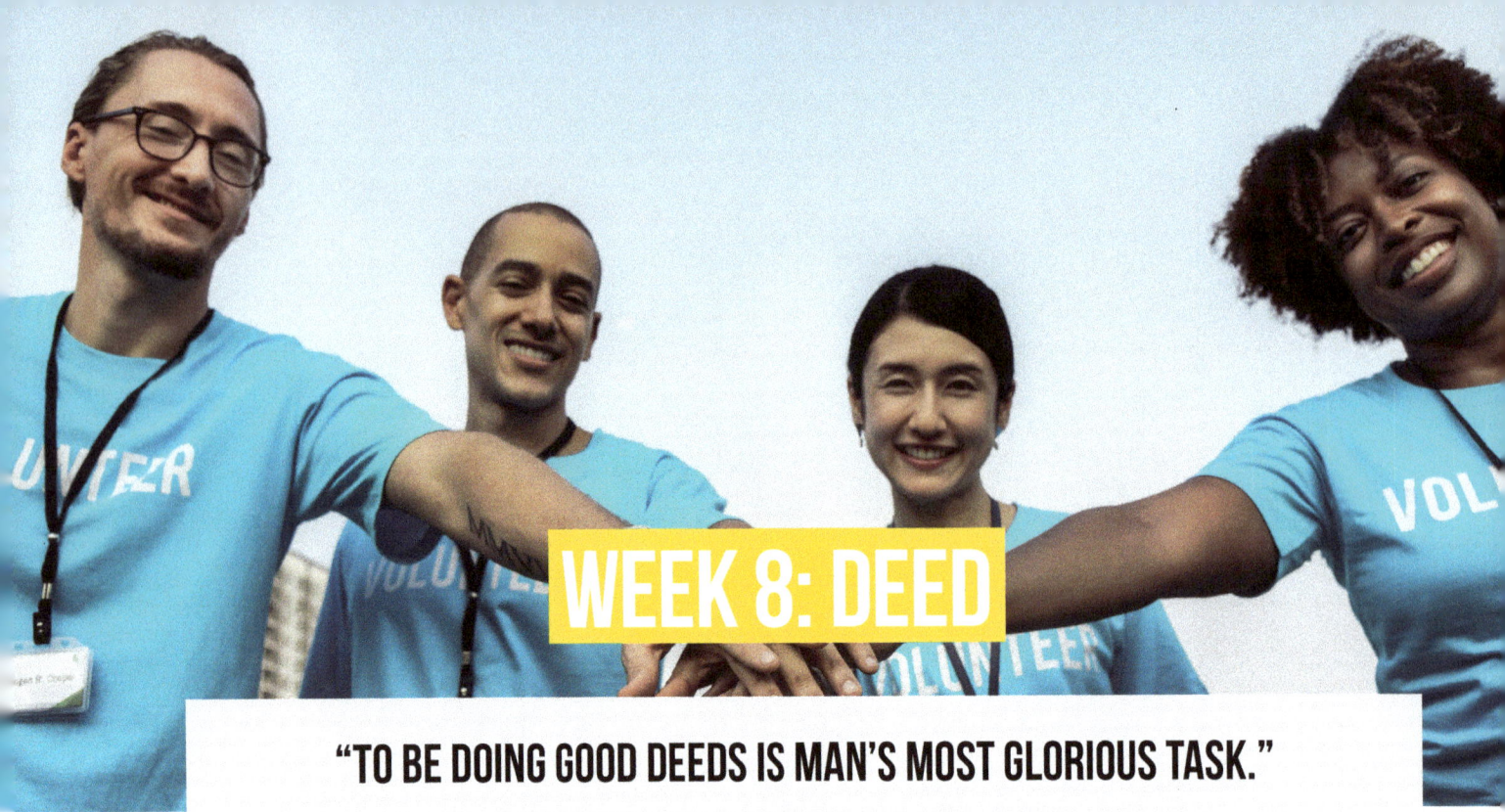

"TO BE DOING GOOD DEEDS IS MAN'S MOST GLORIOUS TASK."

—SOPHOCLES

WEEKLY MENTAL TASK:

Balancing your needs with those of others plays an integral role in your mental well-being. This week, seek out a non-profit organization that promotes a cause you believe in and volunteer at least one hour of your time. Volunteering can be an immensely rewarding experience, and chances are you will gain both new knowledge and new kind-spirited friends in the process!

WEEKLY WORKOUT TASK:

We started slowly with a little bit of stretching in the previous weeks. Now it is time to raise your flexibility game! Choose an area of your body that consistently has limited mobility and apply some tender, loving care. Devote extra time this week to stretching that area with your Stretch Out Strap. Stretch that specific area to the point of slight discomfort or tightness (not pain), and hold the position for 15–30 seconds. Repeat the stretch three times.

TIP:
IF YOU HAVE REGULAR ACCESS TO A STEAM OR SAUNA ROOM, TAKE THE OPPORTUNITY TO COMBINE YOUR SPA SESSION WITH SOME DEEP STRETCHING.

Skip the dessert and treat yourself and your family to a nutrient-dense, health-boosting smoothie instead!

DR. TRINA'S HEALTH-BOOSTING SMOOTHIE

Makes 1 large serving

INGREDIENTS*

- 1/2 thumb-sized turmeric root, peeled
- 1/2 thumb-sized ginger root, peeled
- 1/2 to 3/4 cup unsweetened vanilla almond coconut milk
- 1–2 pitted dates
- 1/4–1/2 cup frozen blueberries
- 1/4 cup fresh pineapple
- 1/2 cup kale
- 1/2 cup bok choy
- 1/2 avocado
- 1/2 banana
- 1/8 cup pumpkin seeds
- 1/4 cup crushed ice

Use organic ingredients if possible.
You can substitute ground turmeric and ginger.

INSTRUCTIONS

Place all ingredients in a blender and blend until smooth. Add a date or 1–2 pineapple chunks if not sweet enough. Pour the contents into a glass and enjoy!

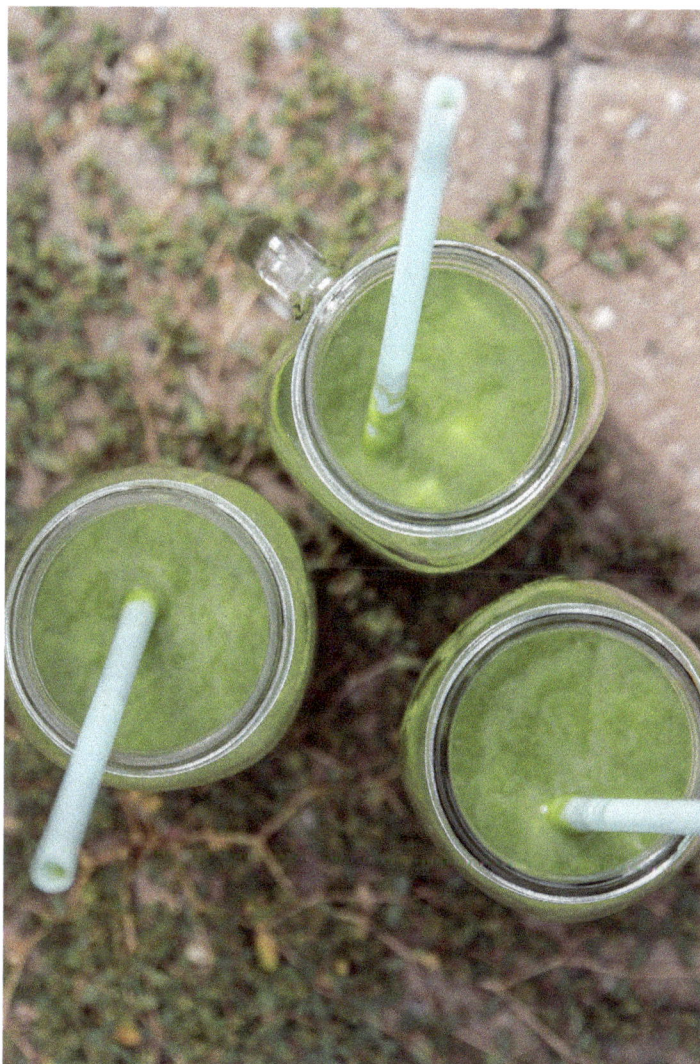

WEEK 9: D VITAMIN

> "SUNSHINE WILL GUIDE YOUR HEART EVEN ON THE MOST DARKEST OF DAYS."
>
> —ANTHONY T. HINCKS

WEEKLY MENTAL TASK:

Few things in life are as healing as being present in the greatness of nature. Take at least 10 minutes daily to sit outside in the sun to soak up some vitamin D. (Make sure to wear sunscreen!) Vitamin D deficiency is common, especially among the elderly and people with dark skin. Sunlight is a great non-dietary source of vitamin D. This vitamin is crucial for proper absorption of calcium, magnesium, and phosphate, as well as the health of several vital body systems (musculoskeletal, nervous, immune, and hormonal). Vitamin D may also play a critical role in defending the body against chronic disease and cancer.

TIP:

MAKE THE MOST OF YOUR TIME IN NATURE AND PRACTICE MINDFUL MEDITATION WHILE YOU SOAK UP THE SUN.

WEEKLY WORKOUT TASK:

Just like vitamin D, strength training is essential to building strong bones. Focus on incorporating strength-building exercises such as push-ups, tricep dips, planks, squats, and lunges. Use your Fit Simplify resistance bands to enhance your training. (See Chapter 18.)

WEEKLY NUTRITION TASK:

Eat more meals rich in vitamin D! Vitamin D is abundant in animal products such as fortified milk and dairy products, salmon, tuna, and sardines. There are also some vegan-friendly vitamin D food sources: mushrooms exposed to sunlight and vitamin D fortified products such as cereal, orange juice, almond milk, rice milk, and soymilk.

WEEK 10: DIARIZE

"YOU CONTROL YOUR FUTURE, YOUR DESTINY. WHAT YOU THINK ABOUT COMES ABOUT. BY RECORDING YOUR DREAMS AND GOALS ON PAPER, YOU SET IN MOTION THE PROCESS OF BECOMING THE PERSON YOU MOST WANT TO BE. PUT YOUR FUTURE IN GOOD HANDS—YOUR OWN."

—MARK VICTOR HANSEN

WEEKLY MENTAL TASK:

Keeping a gratitude journal is a great way to increase positive energy and remind yourself of the progress you have made. Take a few minutes each day—for example, first thing in the morning or right before bed—to record all of the things that make you feel grateful. Your journal can include gratitude for having functional body parts (like having two legs and good eyesight). It can also consist of victories in your nutrition regimen (like keeping your daily sodium intake less than 2,300 mg). Keep in mind that all progress deserves your acknowledgment, no matter how insignificant it may seem!

TIP:

IF YOU HAVE NOT ALREADY DONE SO, TAKE 15 MINUTES TO WRITE DOWN YOUR GOALS, DREAMS, AND PLANS TO ACHIEVE THEM ALONG WITH A TIMETABLE. ONE TRICK FOR SETTING GOALS IS TO FOLLOW THE S.M.A.R.T. MODEL, WHICH STANDS FOR MAKING YOUR GOALS SPECIFIC, MEASURABLE, ASSIGNABLE, REALISTIC, AND TIME-RELATED.

WEEKLY WORKOUT TASK:

While you are getting used to the habit of keeping a gratitude journal, start a workout diary as well! Record your overall fitness and sports activity progress in a separate notebook. Write down all of the physical tasks in which your performance improved and note which tasks need extra attention. Figure out and record how many calories you burned by walking up the stairs. Remember to multiply each stair step by 0.1! Keeping track of your activities will motivate you to push harder and remind you that you are making progress towards your goals.

WEEKLY NUTRITION TASK:

Start keeping a food diary alongside your fitness notebook. Writing down the meals you had in a day will help you gauge how much and what kind of energy you consumed as it relates to your energy expenditure. You will improve your workout results and avoid the unnecessary frustration that comes with stalled progress.

TIP:

HOW MANY NUTRIENT-DENSE MEALS AND SUPERFOODS DID YOU EAT THIS WEEK? HEALTHY NUTRITION IS ABOUT EATING THE RIGHT AMOUNT OF MACRONUTRIENTS (CARBS, FATS, AND PROTEINS) AND THE NECESSARY MICRONUTRIENTS (VITAMINS AND MINERALS)! CHECK HOW MANY MACRONUTRIENTS AND MICRONUTRIENTS YOU HAVE EATEN EACH DAY BY ENTERING YOUR MEALS IN A FREE SMARTPHONE APP LIKE "LOSEIT" OR "MY FITNESSPAL." ONCE YOU GET THE HANG OF THE APPS, THEY CAN BE A TOTAL GAMECHANGER!

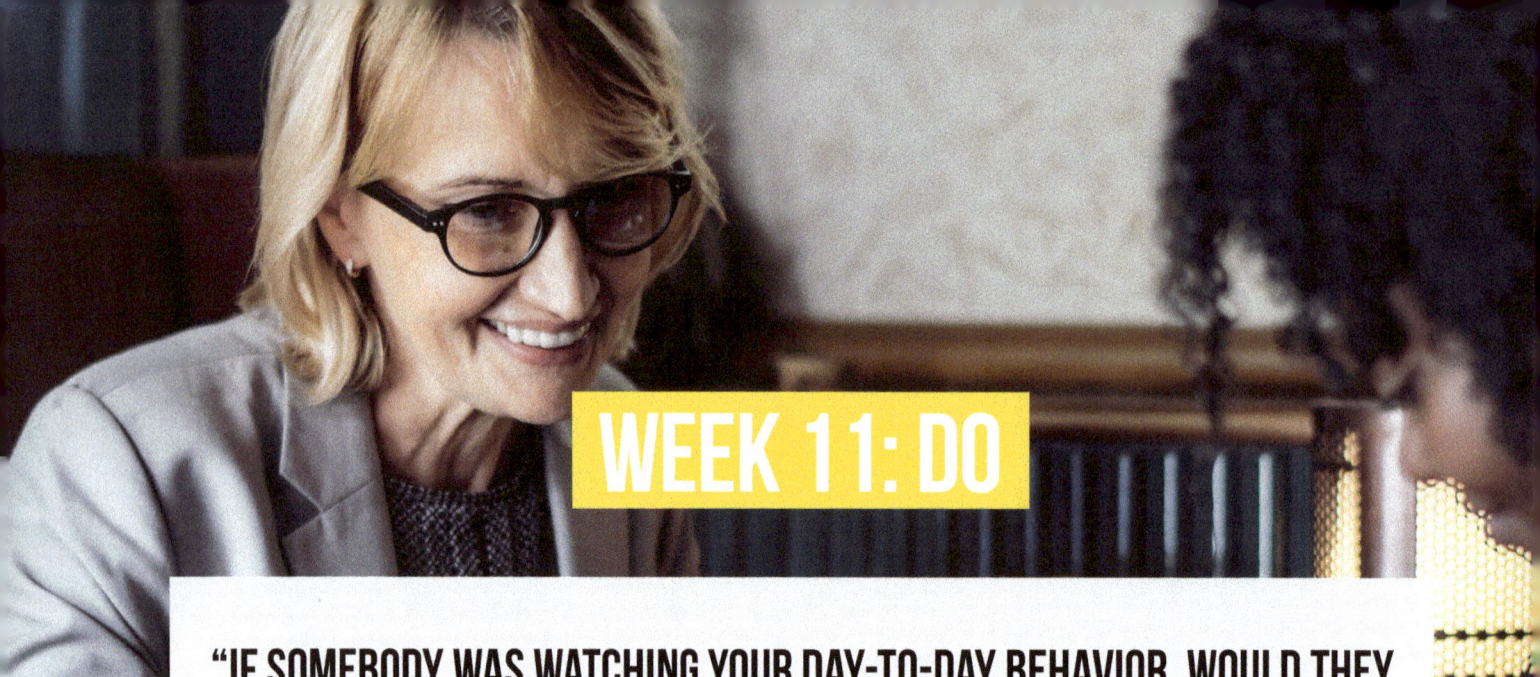

> "IF SOMEBODY WAS WATCHING YOUR DAY-TO-DAY BEHAVIOR, WOULD THEY BE ABLE TO SEE WHAT YOU'RE WORKING TOWARDS, WHAT YOUR GOALS ARE? IF THE ANSWER IS NO, FIX IT!"
>
> —STEVE MARABOLI

WEEKLY MENTAL TASK:

Find a reliable partner to hold you accountable and ask him/her to sign a contract with you that states your commitment to your new healthy lifestyle. Having someone to count on and turn to when you lose motivation or feel lost can be helpful. You may even find that it strengthens your relationship! Many people socialize over gossip and problems instead of having uplifting and energizing conversations. Bonding over inspirational talk is much more conducive to a positive and long-lasting friendship.

Sincerely evaluating the quality of your current relationships can be a significant step towards improving your life. When you realize your true self-worth, you quickly realize that you need to be selective about who you allow in your social circle. You will then automatically attract the right kind of people and enhance your mental well-being.

TIP:

HAVE YOUR ACCOUNTABILITY PARTNER CREATE AN AUDIO RECORDING GIVING YOU A PEP TALK (AND VICE VERSA) FOR WHEN YOU NEED SOME EXTRA ENCOURAGEMENT.

WEEKLY WORKOUT TASK:

Once you begin your chosen sport or physical activity, start practicing the necessary skills to achieve proficiency. When you have learned a skill, the next step is to begin deliberate, focused training to master the skill. Try to perform this skill three times in a row without making an error. If you mess up, you must start over. Over time, aim to perform this skill five times in a row and eventually try ten times in a row without making a mistake. It is incredible how far you can get by pairing simple goals with even the smallest daily commitment!

WEEKLY NUTRITION TASK:

If you are not vegan, challenge yourself to eat only plant-based foods for one week. Record how you feel and evaluate the benefits once the week is over. You may never want to go back! If you already consume a vegan diet, commit to another positive change for the week, such as eating nothing but organic produce, reducing salt intake, eliminating alcohol, or getting rid of processed sugar.

TIP:

FOR WOMEN, DO NOT EXCEED 6 TSP OF SUGAR PER DAY. FOR MEN, DO NOT EXCEED 9 TSP OF SUGAR PER DAY. LIMIT YOUR SODIUM INTAKE TO 1 TSP OR 2300 MG PER DAY. IF YOU ARE IN THE HIGH-RISK GROUP AS MENTIONED IN CHAPTER 8, LIMIT YOUR SODIUM INTAKE TO 3/4 TSP OR 1500 MG.

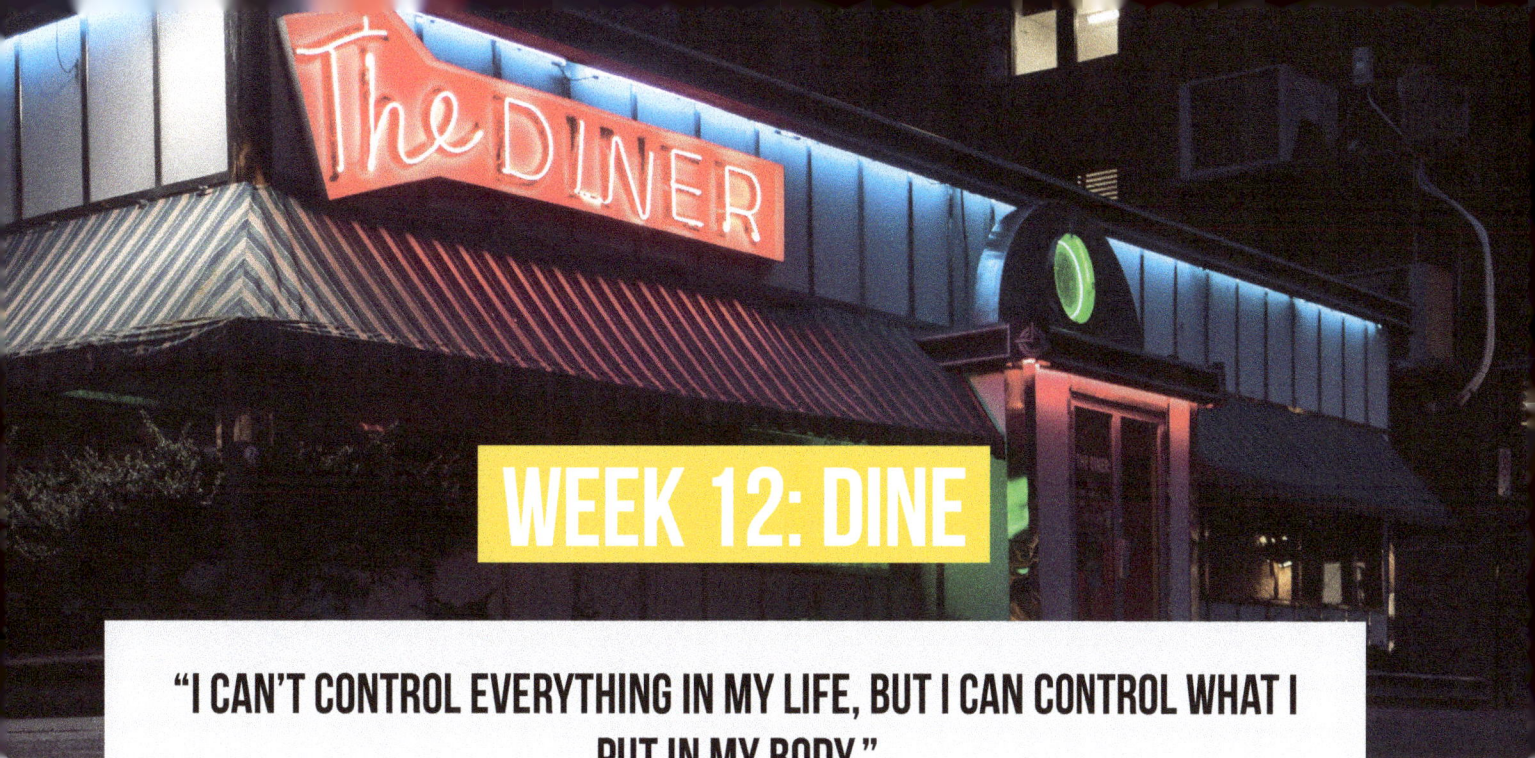

WEEK 12: DINE

> **"I CAN'T CONTROL EVERYTHING IN MY LIFE, BUT I CAN CONTROL WHAT I PUT IN MY BODY."**
>
> — UNKNOWN

WEEKLY MENTAL TASK:

To consistently maintain a healthy diet, you must balance making wise nutrition choices with enjoying the good things in life. Instead of declining that lunch or dinner invitation, make a conscious decision that you will only pick healthy restaurants and meals when you dine out. If you accept an invitation and do not have a say in choosing the restaurant, check the menu online beforehand to evaluate healthy options. Knowing what you will order before you arrive reduces the chance you will succumb to a poor food choice when hunger strikes or when you are rushed to make a quick decision by impatient dining companions.

TIP:

TRY USING THE "HAPPYCOW" APP TO SEARCH FOR HEALTHY RESTAURANTS IN YOUR ZIPCODE.

WEEKLY WORKOUT TASK:

After dining at your new healthy restaurant, reward your body with an invigorating 20–30 minute walk with your dining partner(s)!

WEEKLY NUTRITION TASK:

Progress is about leaving your comfort zone, so don't be afraid to try new things. To avoid remaining a creature of old habits, try at least one new healthy food each day this week.

If you find yourself lacking imagination or inspiration, go to Whole Foods' prepared foods department and ask for samples of healthy dishes you've never tried before. Expand your taste buds with bold choices and do not give up after one or two tries. Keep in mind that it typically takes 3 weeks for your taste buds to acclimate to a new flavor.

TIP:

CONSIDER HIRING A CHEF WHO CAN TEACH YOU HOW TO PREPARE HEALTHY, DELICIOUS MEALS TO GET YOU ON TRACK. IF THAT ISN'T IN YOUR BUDGET, FIND YOUTUBE CHANNELS THAT FOCUS ON CREATING SIMPLE HEALTHY MEALS, SUCH AS SWEET POTATO SOUL, THE DOMESTIC GREEK, TISH WONDERS, CAITLIN SHOEMAKER, CLEAN & DELICIOUS, AND RACHEL AMA.

APPENDIX

— PANTRY MAKEOVER

Out with the old and in with the new! It's time to clear out all overly processed items and make room for nutritious, all-natural health foods.

The list below shows my recommendations for each food category. I've included some of my favorite brands for some products, but feel free to explore your options to find out what you like best.

DRY GOODS

- Organic all-purpose whole wheat flour, whole grain flour

- Natural sweeteners (organic honey, Stevia, Big Tree Farms Organic Brown Coconut Sugar [Unrefined and Low Glycemic Index])

- Steel Cut Oats (Bob's Red Mill Organic Steel Cut Oats)

- Rolled oats (Nature's Path Organic Quick Cook Instant Oats)

- Cornmeal (Bob's Red Mill Cornmeal)

- Baking powder (Hain Pure Foods Baking Powder, Sodium Free and Gluten Free; Rumford Reduced Sodium Aluminum Free Baking Powder)

- Dry beans (black, white, kidney, garbanzo)

- Beans in a carton (Whole Foods' 365 Organic Beans, No Salt Added)

- Organic lentils

- Pasta (Tinkyáda Pasta Joy Brown Rice Pasta; DeLallo Organic Whole-Wheat Pasta; Jovial Organic Brown Rice Pasta; Trader Joe's Organic Whole Wheat Pasta)

- Arrowroot powder for thickening broths (Bob's Red Mill Arrowroot Starch/Flour)

- Yellow corn grits or polenta for more fiber than white grits (Bob's Red Mill Yellow Corn Grits/Polenta)

- Egg replacer (Bob's Red Mill Egg Replacer; Ener-G Egg Replacer; Flax egg: 1 tbsp. flaxseed meal + 2 1/2 tbsp. water)

- Brown rice (Trader Joe's Quick-Cook Organic Brown Basmati Rice; Lundberg Family Farms Organic Black Pearl Rice, Organic California Brown Jasmine Rice, Organic California Brown Basmati Rice)

- Whole-grain bread (Food for Life Ezekiel 4:9 Cinnamon Raisin bread, Angelic Bake House Sprouted Whole Grain and Reduced Sodium, Dave's Killer Bread Thin Sliced 21 Whole Grains and Seeds, Dave's Killer Organic Powerseed Bread)

SAUCES AND OILS

Use sparingly and do not exceed one serving.

- Organic extra virgin olive oil
- Vinegar (Bragg Organic Apple Cider Vinegar)
- Brown rice vinegar (Eden Organic Brown Rice Vinegar)
- Worcestershire sauce (Annie's Organic Vegan Worcestershire Sauce)
- Mustard (365 Organic Yellow Mustard, 365 Organic Dijon Mustard)
- Mayonnaise (Follow Your Heart Soy-Free Vegenaise and Chipotle Vegenaise, Trader Joe's Vegan Spread & Dressing)
- Soy sauce alternative (Bragg Liquid Aminos All Purpose Seasoning)
- Organic, minced garlic (Spice World Organic)
- Ketchup (Annie's Organic Ketchup, Sprouts Farmers Market Reduced Sugar and Sodium Ketchup)
- Barbecue sauce (Annie's Organic Smoky Maple BBQ Sauce, Stevia Sweet Barbecue Sauce)
- Salad dressing (Trader Joe's Almond Butter Turmeric Salad Dressing—located in the cold section; Annie's Balsamic Vinaigrette; Farmer Boy Balsamic Vinaigrette from healthyheartmarket.com; Tessemae's Pantry Classic Balsamic from Sprouts Farmers Market)
- Organic low-sodium vegetable broth (Sprouts Organic Vegetable Broth, Low Sodium)
- Colgin Liquid Smoke (use sparingly)
- Almond butter (Sprouts Organic Unsalted & Unsweetened Creamy Almond Butter)

SPICES

- Basil
- Oregano
- Thyme
- Cumin
- Crushed red pepper
- Cayenne pepper
- Smoked paprika
- Cinnamon
- Curry powder
- Chili powder
- Garlic powder
- Kirkland Signature Organic No-Salt Seasoning
- Rosemary
- Onion powder
- Turmeric
- LoSalt The Original
- Salt-free poultry seasoning
- Salt-free garlic pepper
- Salt-free Italian seasoning
- Salt-free Jamaican jerk
- Salt-free fajita seasoning
- Salt-free Mexican seasoning
- Salt-free lemon pepper
- Salt-free pumpkin spice
- Simply Organic All-Purpose Seasoning
- Vanilla extract

TIP:

SPICE HUNTER, SPROUTS, AND SIMPLY ORGANIC HAVE A VARIETY OF SALT-FREE SEASONINGS.

DAIRY

- Nondairy almond milk (Blue Diamond Almond Breeze Unsweetened Vanilla or Original Almondmilk)

- Nondairy rice milk (Rice Dream Unsweetened Vanilla or Original Rice Drink)

- Butter (Earth Balance Soy Free Buttery Spread; Earth Balance Olive Oil Buttery Spread)

- Nondairy cheese (So Delicious or Daiya Cheddar, Mozzarella, Cheddar-Jack, and Pepperjack)

- Grated parmesan (Parma! Vegan Parmesan)

- Nondairy yogurt (So Delicious Coconutmilk Yogurt; Amande Cultured Almondmilk Yogurt; ; Forager Project Organic Dairy-free Cashewmilk Yogurt, Unsweetened Plain; watch for added sugars)

MEAT ALTERNATIVES

Use occasionally due to increased sodium and saturated fat content.

- Beyond Meat Crumbles and Beyond Meat Hot Italian Sausage (soy-free, GMO-free, cholesterol-free)

- Lightlife Organic Smoky Tempeh Strips

- Soy chorizo (high sodium; use sparingly)

- Jackfruit (It has a shredded, pork-like texture that assumes the flavor of your seasonings. It is also low in sodium and high in fiber.) The Jackfruit Company makes a pre-seasoned jackfruit brand.

- Fresh organic jackfruit (in the produce section at a natural foods market)

- Yves Veggie Pepperoni (not soy-free; use sparingly)

- Gardein Home Style Beefless Tips (not soy-free; use sparingly)

- Veggie burgers (Amy's Organic California Veggie Burger Light in Sodium; dairy-free, soy-free, vegan)

- Field Roast Mexican Chipotle Sausage (vegan, cholesterol-free; high sodium; use sparingly)

- Hilary's Organic Meatless Breakfast Sausage

- Hilary's Grain-Free Super Cauliflower Veggie Burgers

FROZEN FOODS

- Mixed berries (blueberries, acai berries, strawberries, blackberries)
- Cherries
- Pomegranate
- Peaches
- Pineapple (I prefer fresh-cut pineapple for smoothies)
- Edamame
- Organic kale
- Organic spinach
- Amy's Light in Sodium and Non-Dairy Organic Burritos
- Strong Roots Cauliflower Hash Browns

TIP:
USE BANANAS TO MAKE YOUR SMOOTHIES, AND REMEMBER TO FREEZE THEM TO MAKE THEM LAST LONGER. USE FRESH-CUT PINEAPPLE WITH YOUR SMOOTHIES FOR A RICHER TASTE. ADD CRUSHED ICE TO MAKE THE SMOOTHIE COLD AND REFRESHING.

BEVERAGES

Do not drink any store-bought soda or other sugary drinks, and minimize alcohol.

- Alkaline water with electrolytes, such as Essentia
- Sparkling water
- Homemade soda with favorite 100% fruit juice (1/2 cup juice and 1/2 cup sparkling water or 1/4 cup juice and 3/4 cup sparkling water)

DR. TRINA'S FAVORITE TREATS

These snacks are healthier alternatives to occasional treats; use moderately in regard to frequency and serving size.

- Garden of Eatin' Blue Corn Tortilla Chips No Salt Added or Trader Joe's Unsalted Organic White Corn Tortilla Chips served with homemade guacamole
- Late July Snacks' Organic Chia and Quinoa Restaurant Style Tortilla Chips
- Frozen edamame marinated in garlic
- Lenny and Larry's Chocolate Chip Complete Cookie or Whole Foods Vegan Chocolate Chip Cookie
- Almond or cashew dairy-free ice cream
- Whole Foods Vegan Blueberry Muffin

SUPPLEMENTS

Disclaimer: The following list only states my personal supplement preferences and is not to be confused with individual medical advice. To find out if you have any specific vitamin or mineral deficiencies that require a particular supplement regimen, ask your doctor for the appropriate blood tests.

VITAMINS

- Garden of Life Multivitamin (Certified Organic Whole Food)
- Garden of Life Vegan Vitamin D3 (Certified Organic Whole Food)*
- Country Life or Now brand's methyl B-12*

* Vitamin D3 and Vitamin B12 are important if you are vegan.

SUPERFOODS

My top superfoods are turmeric root, ginger root, garlic, Matcha green tea, beets / beetroot powder, flaxseeds, and chia seeds. These superfoods have anti-inflammatory, antioxidant, and anti-cancer properties.

Organic Turmeric and Ginger

You can mix turmeric and ginger in your smoothie. Ginger and turmeric are potent, so do not use too much! For turmeric and ginger, peel off the skin and use about 1/2 length of your index finger. You can also purchase organic ground turmeric and ginger in the spice section of your grocery store.

Matcha green tea

Matcha green tea comes in a powder form and can be consumed as a tea or added to smoothies.

Garlic

Adding garlic to smoothies is not recommended due to its overpowering aftertaste. Instead, I add garlic to my food every day and eat roasted garlic from the olive bars at Whole Foods and Sprouts. Garlic comes in a supplement as well; I prefer Nature's Way brand.

Beets and Beetroot powder

I mix BeetElite by HumanN beetroot powder with water as directed. I also eat roasted beets on a mixed green salad. Beets can enhance energy and performance, support circulation, and lower blood pressure.

Chia Seeds and Flaxseeds

These two superfoods contain essential fatty acids that support your brain, heart, joints, skin, and vision. These little seeds are also great for your digestive health because of their high fiber content. Mix them into your oatmeal or smoothies with superfruits like berries for a significant boost of both omega-3s and antioxidant-rich nutrients! I prefer Spectrum Organic Chia Seeds and Spectrum Organic Ground Flaxseed.

ON THE HORIZON: THE MICROBIOME

Microbiomes are groups of microorganisms that reside together in a specific environment. Any part of the body that interfaces with the universe has a microbiome; that includes the skin, mouth, eyes, airways, vagina, and gastrointestinal tract. The gastrointestinal tract, also known as the gut, has the largest microbiome in the body. Our bodies have approximately 100 trillion microorganisms, including bacteria, viruses, fungi, and other organisms that live on our skin and within our bodies. This number is ten times the number of human cells in our bodies! Everyone has a unique blend of microorganisms in each of their microbiomes. Each person's past and present environment, diet, and lifestyle determine the composition of their microbiomes. Microbiomes have both good and bad bacteria living together in harmony to maintain health. However, if this delicate balance is altered, health problems can arise. Poor diet, stress, toxins, and medications can disrupt this balance, leading to fewer good bacteria and more harmful bacteria. We rely upon these good or helpful microorganisms to do several things: keep our immune system healthy, aid in digestion, produce vitamins, foster critical interaction with nerve and hormonal cells, and maintain optimal mental health and skin health. To help rebalance your microbiomes, consume probiotics and prebiotics. They can help restore the good bacteria to their proper levels.

Probiotics are microorganisms found in certain foods and supplements that help maintain and replenish good bacteria in the gut. There are a plethora of probiotic supplements on the market. Prebiotics are foods that feed and boost the growth of the probiotic bacteria.

Examples of probiotic food include:

- Greek yogurt (no added sugars), kefir, fermented foods (kimchi, kombucha, olives, pickled beets, sauerkraut, soybeans, miso, tempeh)

Examples of prebiotic foods include:

- Fruits (bananas, apples, watermelon, grapefruit)
- Vegetables (garlic, onions, shallots, leeks, cabbage)
- Legumes (chickpeas, lentils, red kidney beans, soybeans)
- Grains (bran, barley, oats)
- Nuts and seeds (almonds, pistachios, flaxseed)

─ RESOURCES

Meditation Apps
      Calm
      Insight Timer
      Headspace
Workout Tools
      Stretchout Strap
      7-min Workout
      FitSimplify.com
Supplements
      Consumerlab.com
Nutritional Facts and Resources
      MyFitnessPal
      FoodData Central
      HealthyHeartMarket.com
Healthy Dining
      Happycow.net
Chefs and Nutritional Coaches
      Bauman College

MACRONUTRIENTS AND MICRONUTRIENTS

The food we eat must supply our bodies with specific nutritional requirements for us to perform well. These dietary requirements are macronutrients and micronutrients. Macronutrients can be divided even further into proteins, carbohydrates, and fats. Large amounts of these nutrients are needed for the body to flourish. On the other hand, the body requires small amounts of micronutrients (vitamins and minerals) to function properly.

FATS

Fats should account for about 15–20% of your daily calorie intake. They are essential for brain development, cell function, vitamin absorption, and shock absorption for your organs.

Example of good fats: avocado, seeds, nuts, olives, tofu, and fatty fish such as salmon, mackerel, herring, trout, sardines, and albacore tuna

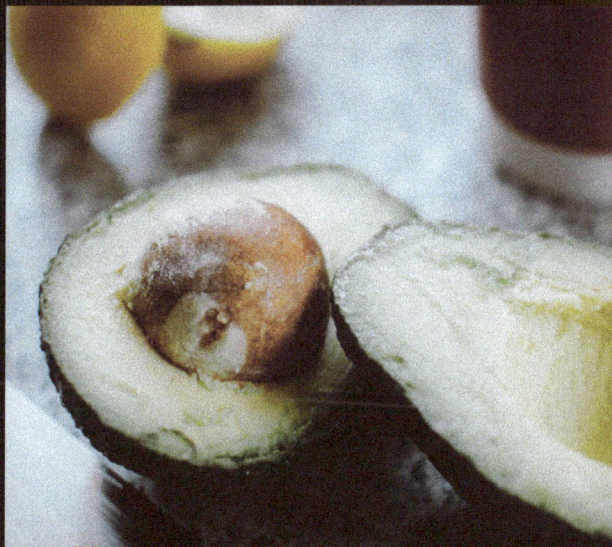

PROTEINS

Proteins, also known as the building blocks of our bodies, should make up 10–35% of our daily calorie intake. They are involved in the repair, regeneration, and maintenance of body tissues and cells.

Examples of protein foods: lean meats, seafood, beans, soy, eggs, nuts, seeds, peanut butter, pumpkin seeds, edamame pods, tofu, Greek yogurt, quinoa, and lentils

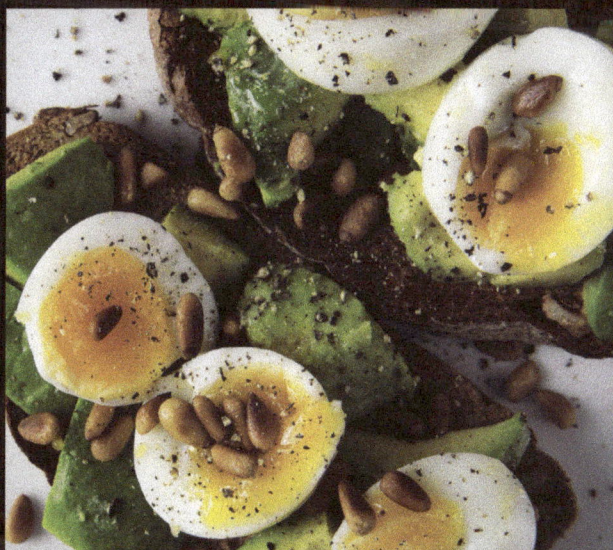

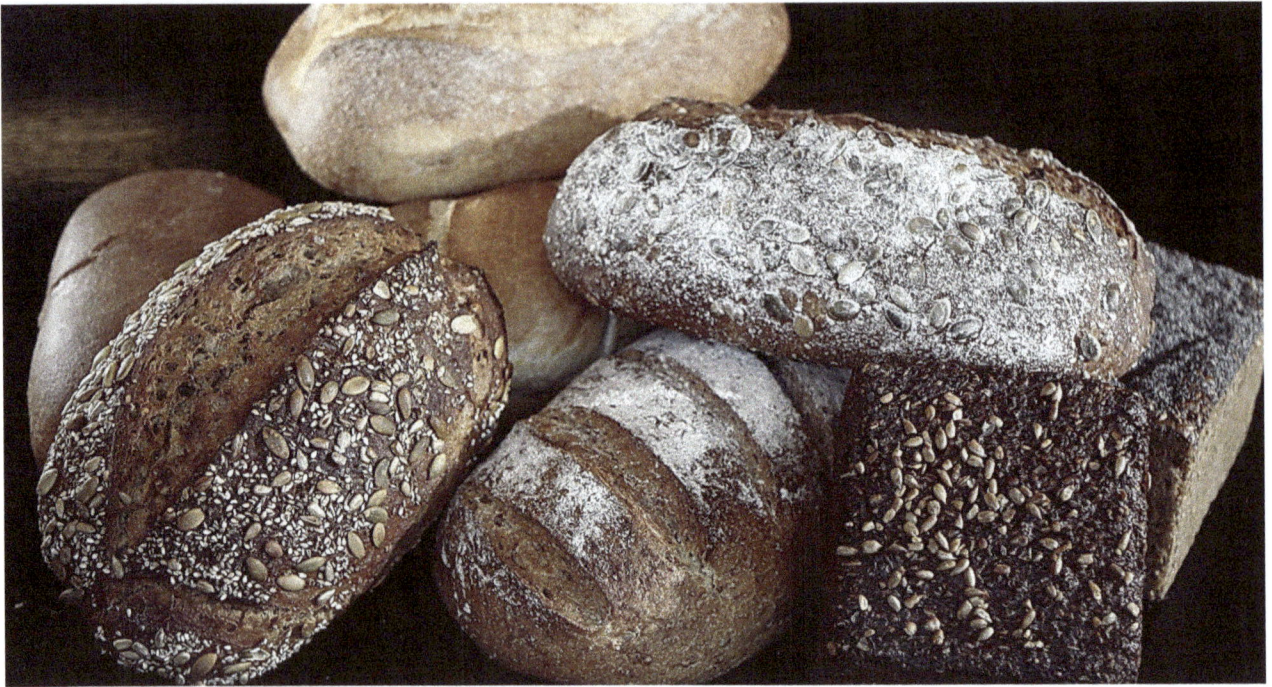

CARBOHYDRATES

Carbohydrates should make up 45–65% of your daily diet. Carbohydrates come in two forms: simple and complex. Complex carbohydrates are comprised of starches and fiber. Only simple carbohydrates and starches can be broken down into glucose, the body's main source of energy. Simple carbohydrates are immediately broken down into sugar, causing spikes in your blood sugar. In contrast, starches are slowly broken down into sugar and produce a more gradual rise in blood sugar and fewer fluctuations. Fiber, on the other hand, is the part of plants that can't be broken down. It passes through the body without being digested. Fiber does several important jobs: lowers cholesterol, removes carcinogenic agents from the body, helps the colon stay healthy, and controls weight.

Examples of simple carbohydrates:
baked goods made with white flour, white sugar, and most packaged cereals

Examples of complex carbohydrates:
100% whole-grain bread, 100% whole-grain flour, 100% whole-grain pasta, yams, sweet potatoes, oatmeal, beans, brown rice, and quinoa

Examples of high-fiber foods:
raspberries, pears, apples, strawberries, green peas, broccoli, turnip and collard greens, Brussels sprouts, all-bran flakes, quinoa, oatmeal, brown rice, 100% whole-wheat bread, legumes, beans, nuts, and seeds

— BIBLIOGRAPHY

Alissa EM, Ferns GA. Dietary fruits, vegetables, and cardiovascular diseases risk. *Crit Rev Food Sci Nutr.* 2017;57(9):1950-1962.

Aridi YS, Walker JL, Wright ORL. The association between the Mediterranean dietary pattern and cognitive health: A systematic review. *Nutrients.* 2017;9(7):674.

Barański M, Srednicka-Tober D, Volakakis N, Seal C, Sanderson R, Stewart GB, Benbrook C, Biavati B, Markellou E, Giotis C, Gromadzka-Ostrowska J, Rembiałkowska E, Skwarło-Sońta K, Tahvonen R, Janovská D, Niggli U, Nicot P, Leifert C. Higher antioxidant and lower cadmium concentrations and lower incidence of pesticide residues in organically grown crops: A systematic literature review and meta-analyses. *Br J Nutr.* 2014;112(5):794-811.

Baudry J, Lelong H, Adriouch S, Julia C, Allès B, Hercberg S, Touvier M, Lairon D, Galan P, Kesse-Guyot E. Association between organic food consumption and metabolic syndrome: Cross-sectional results from the NutriNet-Santé study. *Eur J Nutr.* 2018;57(7):2477-2488.

Cecchini M, Warin L. Impact of food labelling systems on food choices and eating behaviours: A systematic review and meta-analysis of randomized studies. *Obes Rev.* 2016;17(3):201-210.

Chauhan R, Kumari B, Rana MK. Effect of fruit and vegetable processing on reduction of synthetic pyrethroid residues. *Rev Environ Contam Toxicol.* 2014;229:89-110.

Chen Z, Zuurmond MG, van der Schaft N, Nano J, Wijnhoven HAH, Ikram MA, Franco OH, Voortman T. Plant versus animal based diets and insulin resistance, prediabetes and type 2 diabetes: The Rotterdam Study. *Eur J Epidemiol.* 2018;33(9):883-893.

Christoph MJ, An R, Ellison B. Correlates of nutrition label use among college students and young adults: A review. *Public Health Nutr.* 2016;19(12):2135-2148.

Christoph MJ, Ellison BD, Meador EN. The influence of nutrition label placement on awareness and use among college students in a dining hall setting. *J Acad Nutr Diet.* 2016;116(9):1395-1405.

Chung SW. How effective are common household preparations on removing pesticide residues from fruit and vegetables? A review. *J Sci Food Agric.* 2018;98(8):2857-2870.

Clifton PM, Keogh JB. A systematic review of the effect of dietary saturated and polyunsaturated fat on heart disease. *Nutr Metab Cardiovasc Dis.* 2017;27(12):1060- 1080.

Cogswell ME, Zhang Z, Carriquiry AL, Gunn JP, Kuklina EV, Saydah SH, Yang Q, Moshfegh AJ. Sodium and potassium intakes among US adults: NHANES 2003-2008. *Am J Clin Nutr.* 2012;96(3):647-657

Cook NR, Appel LJ, Whelton PK. Sodium intake and all-cause mortality over 20 years in the trials of hypertension prevention. *J Am Coll Cardiol.* 2016;68(15):1609-1617.

Dahl WJ, Stewart ML. Position of the Academy of Nutrition and Dietetics: Health implications of dietary fiber. *J Acad Nutr Diet.* 2015;115(11):1861-1870.

Dinu M, Pagliai G, Sofi F. A heart-healthy diet: recent insights and practical recommendations. Curr *Cardiol Rep.* 2017;19(10):95.

Dolmatova EV, Moazzami K, Bansilal S. Dietary sodium intake among US adults with hypertension, 1999-2012. *J Hypertens.* 2018;36(2):237-242.

Dreher ML. Whole fruits and fruit fiber emerging health effects. *Nutrients.* 2018;10(12):1833.

Duvivier BM, Schaper NC, Hesselink MK, van Kan L, Stienen N, Winkens B, Koster A, Savelberg HH. Breaking sitting with light activities vs structured exercise: A randomised crossover study demonstrating benefits for glycaemic control and insulin sensitivity in type 2 diabetes. *Diabetologia.* 2017;60(3):490-498.

Farha W, Abd El-Aty AM, Rahman MM, Jeong JH, Shin HC, Wang J, Shin SS, Shim JH. Analytical approach, dissipation pattern and risk assessment of pesticide residue in green leafy vegetables: A comprehensive review. *Biomed Chromatogr.* January 2018;32(1):e4134.

Fresán U, Gea A, Bes-Rastrollo M, Ruiz-Canela M, Martínez-Gonzalez MA. Substitution models of water for other beverages, and the incidence of obesity and weight gain in the SUN Cohort. *Nutrients.* 2016;8(11):688.

Friedenreich CM, Shaw E, Neilson HK, Brenner DR. Epidemiology and biology of physical activity and cancer recurrence. *J Mol Med (Berl).* 2017;95(10):1029-1041.

Gould Rothberg BE, Bulloch KJ, Fine JA, Barnhill RL, Berwick M. Red meat and fruit intake is prognostic among patients with localized cutaneous melanomas more than 1mm thick. *Cancer Epidemiol.* 2014;38(5):599-607.

Harnack LJ, Cogswell ME, Shikany JM, Gardner CD, Gillespie C, Loria CM, Zhou X, Yuan K, Steffen LM. Sources of sodium in US adults from 3 geographic regions. *Circulation.* 2017;135(19):1775-1783.

Hawkins MAW, Keirns NG, Helms Z. Carbohydrates and cognitive function. *Curr Opin Clin Nutr Metab Care.* 2018;21(4):302-307.

Johnson RK, Appel LJ, Brands M, Howard BV, Lefevre M, Lustig RH, Sacks F, Steffen LM, Wylie-Rosett J; American Heart Association Nutrition Committee of the Council on Nutrition, Physical Activity, and Metabolism and the Council on Epidemiology and Prevention. Dietary sugars intake and cardiovascular health: A scientific statement from the American Heart Association. *Circulation.* 2009;120(11):1011-1020.

Joseph SV, Edirisinghe I, Burton-Freeman BM. Berries: Anti-inflammatory effects in humans. *J Agric Food Chem.* 2014;62(18):3886-3903.

Khodarahmi M, Azadbakht L. The association between different kinds of fat intake and breast cancer risk in women. *Int J Prev Med*. 2014;5(1):6-15.

Kliemann N, Kraemer MVS, Scapin T, Rodrigues VM, Fernandes AC, Bernardo GL, Uggioni PL, Proença RPC. Serving size and nutrition labelling: Implications for nutrition information and nutrition claims on packaged foods. *Nutrients*. 2018;10(7):891.

Li N, Petrick JL, Steck SE, Bradshaw PT, McClain KM, Niehoff NM, Engel LS, Shaheen NJ, Corley DA, Vaughan TL, Gammon MD. Dietary sugar/starches intake and Barrett's esophagus: A pooled analysis. *Eur J Epidemiol*. 2017;32(11):1007-1017.

Liu AG, Ford NA, Hu FB, Zelman KM, Mozaffarian D, Kris-Etherton PM. A healthy approach to dietary fats: Understanding the science and taking action to reduce consumer confusion. *Nutr J*. 2017;16(1):53.

Mancini E, Beglinger C, Drewe J, Zanchi D, Lang UE, Borgwardt S. Green tea effects on cognition, mood and human brain function: A systematic review. *Phytomedicine*. October 2017;34:26-37.

Mantha M, Yeary E, Trent J, Creed PA, Kubachka K, Hanley T, Shockey N, Heitkemper D, Caruso J, Xue J, Rice G, Wymer L, Creed JT. Estimating inorganic arsenic exposure from U.S. rice and total water intakes. *Environ Health Perspect*. 2017;125(5):057005.

McEvoy CT, Guyer H, Langa KM, Yaffe K. Neuroprotective diets are associated with better cognitive function: The health and retirement study. *J Am Geriatr Soc*. 2017;65(8):1857-1862.

Mie A, Andersen HR, Gunnarsson S, Kahl J, Kesse-Guyot E, Rembiałkowska E, Quaglio G, Grandjean P. Human health implications of organic food and organic agriculture: A comprehensive review. *Environ Health*. 2017;16(1):111.

Miller V, Mente A, Dehghan M, Rangarajan S, Zhang X, Swaminathan S, Dagenais G, Gupta R, Mohan V, Lear S, Bangdiwala SI, Schutte AE, Wentzel-Viljoen E, Avezum A, Altuntas Y, Yusoff K, Ismail N, Peer N, Chifamba J, Diaz R, Rahman O, Mohammadifard N, Lanas F, Zatonska K, Wielgosz A, Yusufali A, Iqbal R, Lopez-Jaramillo P, Khatib R, Rosengren A, Kutty VR, Li W, Liu J, Liu X, Yin L, Teo K, Anand S, Yusuf S; Prospective Urban Rural Epidemiology (PURE) study investigators. Fruit, vegetable, and legume intake, and cardiovascular disease and deaths in 18 countries (PURE): A prospective cohort study. *Lancet*. 2017;390(10107):2037-2049.

Mohan A, Sharma R, Bijlani RL. Effect of meditation on stress-induced changes in cognitive functions. *J Altern Complement Med*. 2011;17(3):207-212.

Moshfegh AJ, Holden JM, Cogswell ME, Kuklina EV, Patel SM, Gunn JP, Gillespie C, Hong Y, Merritt R, Galuska DA; Centers for Disease Control and Prevention (CDC). Vital signs: Food categories contributing the most to sodium consumption—United States, 2007-2008. *MMWR Morb Mortal Wkly Rep*. February 10, 2012;61(5):92-98.

Mostofsky E, Chahal HS, Mukamal KJ, Rimm EB, Mittleman MA. Alcohol and immediate risk of cardiovascular events: A systematic review and dose-response meta-analysis. *Circulation*. 2016;133(10):979-987.

Mozaffarian D, Aro A, Willett WC. Health effects of trans-fatty acids: Experimental and observational evidence. *Eur J Clin Nutr*. 2009;63(suppl 2):S5-21.

Murphy MM, Barraj LM, Spungen JH, Herman DR, Randolph RK. Global assessment of select phytonutrient intakes by level of fruit and vegetable consumption. *Br J Nutr*. 2014;112(6):1004-1018.

New and Improved Nutrition Facts Label. Food and Drug Administration website. https://www.fda.gov/food/nutrition- education-resources-and-materials/new-and-improved-nutrition-facts-label. Updated July 6, 2018. Accessed May 17, 2019.

Orkaby AR, Forman DE. Physical activity and CVD in older adults: An expert's perspective. *Expert Rev Cardiovasc Ther*. 2018;16(1):1-10.

Patel H, Chandra S, Alexander S, Soble J, Williams KA Sr. Plant-based nutrition: An essential component of cardiovascular disease prevention and management. *Curr Cardiol Rep*. 2017;19(10):104.

Phillips C. Lifestyle modulators of neuroplasticity: How physical activity, mental engagement, and diet promote cognitive health during aging. *Neural Plast*. 2017;2017:3589271.

Pollock RL. The effect of green leafy and cruciferous vegetable intake on the incidence of cardiovascular disease: A meta-analysis. *JRSM Cardiovasc Dis*. 2016;5. doi: 10.1177/2048004016661435.

Price CT, Langford JR, Liporace FA. Essential nutrients for bone health and a review of their availability in the average North American diet. *Open Orthop J*. 2012;6:143-149.

Ratna A, Mandrekar P. Alcohol and cancer: Mechanisms and therapies. *Biomolecules*. 2017;7(3):61.

Sacks M. Why dance matters. *Stanford*. May 2019. https://stanfordmag.org/contents/why-dance-matters. Accessed January 16, 2020.

Satija A, Bhupathiraju SN, Rimm EB, Spiegelman D, Chiuve SE, Borgi L, Willett WC, Manson JE, Sun Q, Hu FB. Plant-based dietary patterns and incidence of type 2 diabetes in US men and women: Results from three prospective cohort studies. *PLoS Med*. 2016;13(6):e1002039.

Schlesinger S, Neuenschwander M, Schwedhelm C, Hoffmann G, Bechthold A, Boeing H, Schwingshackl L. Food groups and risk of overweight, obesity, and weight gain: A systematic review and dose-response meta-analysis of prospective studies. *Adv Nutr*. 2019;10(2):205-218.

Scrivo R, Perricone C, Altobelli A, Castellani C, Tinti L, Conti F, Valesini G. Dietary habits bursting into the complex pathogenesis of autoimmune diseases: The emerging role of salt from experimental and clinical studies. *Nutrients*. 2019;11(5):1013.

Shangguan S, Afshin A, Shulkin M, Ma W, Marsden D, Smith J, Saheb-Kashaf M, Shi P, Micha R, Imamura F, Mozaffarian D; Food PRICE (Policy Review and Intervention Cost-Effectiveness) Project. A meta-analysis of food labeling effects on consumer diet behaviors and industry practices. *Am J Prev Med*. 2019;56(2):300-314.

Tanabe CK, Nelson J, Ebeler SE. Current perspective on arsenic in wines: Analysis, speciation, and changes in composition during production. *J Agric Food Chem*. 2019;67(15):4154-4159.

Traversy G, Chaput JP. Alcohol consumption and obesity: An update. *Curr Obes Rep*. 2015;4(1):122-130.

Wanders AJ, Zock PL, Brouwer IA. Trans fat intake and its dietary sources in general populations worldwide: A systematic review. *Nutrients*. 2017;9(8):840.

Wesselman LMP, Doorduijn AS, de Leeuw FA, Verfaillie SCJ, van Leeuwenstijn-Koopman M, Slot RER, Kester MI, Prins ND, van de Rest O, de van der Schueren MAE, Scheltens P, Sikkes SAM, van der Flier WM. Dietary patterns are related to clinical characteristics in memory clinic patients with subjective cognitive decline: The SCIENCe Project. *Nutrients*. 2019;11(5):1057.

Yang Q, Liu T, Kuklina EV, Flanders WD, Hong Y, Gillespie C, Chang MH, Gwinn M, Dowling N, Khoury MJ, Hu FB. Sodium and potassium intake and mortality among US adults: Prospective data from the Third National Health and Nutrition Examination Survey. *Arch Intern Med*. 2011;171(13):1183-1191.

― REFERENCES

p13   1. The 10-20-30 training concept improves performance and health profile in moderately trained runners
https://www.physiology.org/doi/full/10.1152/japplphysiol.00334.2012

p31   1. Dietary Guidelines Advisory Committee Recommedations
https://www.dietaryguidelines.gov/sites/default/files/2020-12/Dietary_Guidelines_for_Americans_2020-2025.pdf

p35   1. Red and processed meat and colorectal cancer incidence: meta-analysis of prospective studies
https://www.ncbi.nlm.nih.gov/pubmed/21674008

p39   1. Alcohol consumption as a cause of cancer
https://onlinelibrary.wiley.com/doi/abs/10.1111/add.13477

   2. 2018 study on alcohol consumption
https://www.thelancet.com/article/S0140-6736(18)31571-X/fulltext

p40   1. Ultra-Processed Food Consumption and Chronic Non-Communicable Diseases-Related Dietary Nutrient Profile in the UK (2008–2014)
https://www.ncbi.nlm.nih.gov/pmc/articles/PMC5986467/

   2. Food Consumption and its impact on Cardiovascular Disease: Importance of Solutions focused on the globalized food system
https://www.ncbi.nlm.nih.gov/pmc/articles/PMC4597475/

   3. Ultra-processed foods might increase cancer risk
https://www.thelancet.com/journals/lanonc/article/PIIS1470-2045(18)30184-0/fulltext

p47   1. Cancer health effects of pesticides
https://www.ncbi.nlm.nih.gov/pmc/articles/PMC2231435/

   2. Higher PUFA and n-3 PUFA, conjugated linoleic acid, α-tocopherol and iron, but lower iodine and selenium concentrations in organic milk: a systematic literature review and meta- and redundancy analyses.
https://www.ncbi.nlm.nih.gov/pubmed/26878105

   3. Composition differences between organic and conventional meat: a systematic literature review and meta-analysis
https://www.cambridge.org/core/services/aop-cambridge-core/content/view/S0007114515005073

4. Higher antioxidant and lower cadmium concentrations and lower incidence of pesticide residues in organically grown crops: a systematic literature review and meta-analyses.
   https://www.ncbi.nlm.nih.gov/pubmed/24968103

5. Neonicotinoid pesticides can reduce honeybee colony genetic diversity
   https://www.ncbi.nlm.nih.gov/pmc/articles/PMC5653293/

p53
1. Twelve Weeks of Sprint Interval Training Improves Indices of Cardiometabolic Health Similar to Traditional Endurance Training despite a Five-Fold Lower Exercise Volume and Time Commitment
   https://journals.plos.org/plosone/article?id=10.1371/journal.pone.0154075

p55
1. The Impact of Bdnf Gene Deficiency to the Memory Impairment and Brain Pathology of APPswe/PS1dE9 Mouse Model of Alzheimer's Disease
   https://www.ncbi.nlm.nih.gov/pmc/articles/PMC3700921/

2. The Aging Hippocampus: Interactions between Exercise, Depression, and BDNF
   https://www.ncbi.nlm.nih.gov/pmc/articles/PMC3575139/

3. The Effects of Aerobic Exercise Intensity and Duration on Levels of Brain-Derived Neurotrophic Factor in Healthy Men
   https://www.ncbi.nlm.nih.gov/pmc/articles/PMC3772595/

p61
1. Controlled trial of fasting and one-year vegetarian diet in rheumatoid arthritis
   https://www.thelancet.com/journals/lancet/article/PII0140-6736(91)91770-U/fulltext

2. Whole-Foods, Plant-Based Diet Alleviates the Symptoms of Osteoarthritis
   https://www.ncbi.nlm.nih.gov/pmc/articles/PMC4359818/

3. Green tea: a new option for the prevention or control of osteoarthritis
   https://www.ncbi.nlm.nih.gov/pmc/articles/PMC3239363/

4. Association between dietary fiber and serum C-reactive protein
   https://www.ncbi.nlm.nih.gov/pmc/articles/PMC1456807/

p73
1. Effect of meditation on stress-induced changes in cognitive functions.
   https://www.ncbi.nlm.nih.gov/pubmed/21417807

2. Effects of the transcendental meditation technique on trait anxiety: a meta-analysis of randomized controlled trials.
   https://www.ncbi.nlm.nih.gov/pubmed/24107199

3. Relationships between mindfulness practice and levels of mindfulness, medical and psychological symptoms and well-being in a mindfulness-based stress reduction program
https://www.researchgate.net/publication/5946075_Relationships_between_mindfulness_practice_and_levels_of_mindfulness_medical_and_psychological_symptoms_and_well-being_in_a_mindfulness-based_stress_reduction_program

4. Three-year follow-up and clinical implications of a mindfulness meditation-based stress reduction intervention in the treatment of anxiety disorders
https://www.sciencedirect.com/science/article/pii/016383439500025M

5. Effect of meditation on neurophysiological changes in stress mediated depression.
https://www.ncbi.nlm.nih.gov/pubmed/24439650

6. Alterations in Brain and Immune Function Produced by Mindfulness Meditation
https://journals.lww.com/psychosomaticmedicine/Abstract/2003/07000/Alterations_in_Brain_and_Immune_Function_Produced.14.aspx

7. The Effects of School-Based Maum Meditation Program on the Self-Esteem and School Adjustment in Primary School Students
https://www.ncbi.nlm.nih.gov/pmc/articles/PMC4776824/

8. Attention regulation and monitoring in meditation
https://www.ncbi.nlm.nih.gov/pmc/articles/PMC2693206/

9. Mindfulness meditation as an intervention for binge eating, emotional eating, and weight loss: a systematic review.
https://www.ncbi.nlm.nih.gov/pubmed/24854804

10. A Narrative Review of Yoga and Mindfulness as Complementary Therapies for Addiction
https://www.ncbi.nlm.nih.gov/pmc/articles/PMC3646290/

p84

1. Essential oil of lavender in anxiety disorders: Ready for prime time?
https://www.ncbi.nlm.nih.gov/pmc/articles/PMC6007527/

2. Lavender and the Nervous System
https://www.ncbi.nlm.nih.gov/pmc/articles/PMC3612440/